DO NO HARM:
FATPHOBIA AND
THE MEDICAL INDUSTRY

DO NO HARM:

FATPHOBIA AND
THE MEDICAL INDUSTRY

HANNAH HAWKINS

NEW DEGREE PRESS

DO NO HARM:

Fatphobia and the Medical Industry

ISBN   978-1-63676-557-0 *Paperback*

            978-1-63676-136-7 *Kindle Ebook*

            978-1-63676-137-4 *Ebook*

CONTENTS

———

ACKNOWLEDGMENTS   7

INTRODUCTION   11

ACKNOWLEDGING MY PRIVILEGE   19

INSPIRATION STORY   23

PART 1.   **WHEN AND HOW DID SOCIETY BECOME SO FATPHOBIC?**   **27**

CHAPTER 1.   DIET CULTURE'S HEAVY HAND   29

CHAPTER 2.   RACISM, FATPHOBIA, AND ITS IMPACT ON THE "O WORD" EPIDEMIC   51

CHAPTER 3.   WHY WEIGHT LOSS ISN'T SUSTAINABLE: BIGGEST LOSER STUDY   71

PART 2.   **HOW FATPHOBIA IS MARGINALIZING PEOPLE AND HARMING SOCIETY**   **77**

CHAPTER 4.   FATPHOBIA AND HEALTH CARE AVOIDANCE   79

CHAPTER 5.   FATPHOBIA AND LATE DIAGNOSES   95

CHAPTER 6.   EMPLOYERS, INSURANCE COVERAGE, AND FATPHOBIA   103

CHAPTER 7.   FATPHOBIA AND QUACK DOCTORS   115

CHAPTER 8.   CHILDREN AND FATPHOBIA   125

CHAPTER 9.   THE DANGERS OF GASTRIC BYPASS SURGERY   143

PART 3. **ADVOCATING FOR YOURSELF,**
DISROBING YOUR OWN FATPHOBIA,
AND PRACTICING WEIGHT-INCLUSIVE
MEDICINE **151**

CHAPTER 10. HAES AND WHY IT WORKS 153

CHAPTER 11. WHY ALL DOCTORS SHOULD DITCH
"WEIGHT MANAGEMENT" METHODS AND
ADOPT INTUITIVE EATING AS HEALTH
INTERVENTION 165

CHAPTER 12. WEIGHT MANAGEMENT HAS NO PLACE
IN EVIDENCE-BASED CARE 171

CHAPTER 13. STORIES FROM THE DOCTOR'S OFFICE:
HOW THESE WOMEN ADVOCATED FOR
THEMSELVES 185

CONCLUSION 197

APPENDIX 201

ACKNOWLEDGMENTS

Addis Sansone
Alanis Koberlein
Alexis Gautier
Aliyah Adams
Alyssa Kohler
Alyssa Mossotti
Amanda Miller
Amber Kesterson
Amy Maurer
Andrew Entrikin
Andrew Gonzales
Angie Pulley
Anna Marie Wright
Anne K Patterson
Annie Day
Annie Goldsmith
Annie Mohr
Ashleigh Smith
Ashley Ferraro
Ashlynn Cetera
Barbara Srnovrsnik

Beth Donlon
Bethany Carroll
Bill Hoover
Bre Norton
Brooke Bailey
C. & Reeves Towery
Carmen Garmilla
Caroline Lueck
Carrie Kennedy
Chelsea Schmidt
Chloe Johnson
Christina Drogaris
Christine Roper
Cindy Kopff
Claire Chiarotti
Claudia Villegas
Colleen Kane
Daniel Papa
David Leonard
Debra Richter
Denise Gruender

Elise George
Elizabeth Alba
Emily Brinkley
Emily Corsi Shepard
Emily De Aguiar
Emily K Killian
Emily McWey
Eric Koester
Georgia Fontana
Gina Salamie
Greg Mercer
Grier McLaurin
Haley Hawkins
Hannah Hatton
Hannah Taylor
Hunter Kicklighter
Jack & Kim Hawkins
Jacqueline Faerman
Jacqueline Flynn
Jamie Marquis
Jamie Stocker
Jennifer Rutalis
Jodi Seidel
Jonah Baer
Jordan Ernsberger
Jordana McCulloch
Joshua Howard
Juliet Kuehnle
Kaitlin Cash
Karen Buffington
Katherine Martin
Kathleen Cross

Katie Gallagher
Katie Gavlick
Katie Mackoul
Katie Reich
Katie Roca
Kerry Price
Kim Matone
Kimberly Kicklighter
Kimiyo Karosas
Kitty Weaver
Laura Crawford
Laura Grady
Lauren Jackson
Leah Graham
Lexie Cheokas
Lisa Qualtieri
Mackenzie Harty
Maggie Moore
Makenzie Brooks
Maressa Benz
Maria Leal-Bruce
Mariah Shaw
Marissa Ramirez
Mark Hutto
Mary Louise Roam
Maxwell McArthur
Megan Leigh Zban
Megan Richter
Millie Blount
MJ Miller
Molly Brisendine
Molly Ryan

Morgan Martino
Nancy E. Hawkins
Natalie de la Guarda
Natalie Hoover
Niki DuBois
Nkyla Ellerbee
Nora King
Norman George
Olivia DiNome
Omari Prescod
Patricia Robinson
Pierre LeLeux
Rachel Pepper
Rachel Rodriguez
Rachel Stys
Rebecca Stapp
Renee Foster
Rob Sullivan
Rose Rodgers-Dryfoos
Samantha Perkowski

Sandra Chaplin
Sara Cooksey
Sara Sigel
Sarah Griffin
Shaniah Caldwell
Sharon Hartman
Shelby West
Sheridan Hager
Sherrie Andrews
Sonia Kolli
Steven Reisner
Sylvie Grasheim
Taylor Self
Taylor Shaw
Timothy Roche
Tori Monical
Travis Lawrence
Tyler Duval
William Entrikin
Wilshem Pennick

INTRODUCTION

The blistering heat of Los Angeles beat down in summer of 2019, as mother-to-be Jen Curran almost became victim to our fatphobic medical system and could have lost her life. Curran found out at her second trimester OB/GYN appointment that she had high blood pressure and high levels of protein in her urine. She was diagnosed with pre-eclampsia, a pregnancy complication, and "put it out of her mind," then went on bed rest per doctor's orders.

Pre-eclampsia is one of many conditions that has obesity listed as a "high risk factor" for its development, without much evidence to back the claim. Jen fit the description in the doctor's eyes, and not long after giving birth to her daughter Rose, Curran's blood pressure returned to normal, but the protein levels in her urine increased.

Her doctor told her she needed to lose weight to get her protein levels back to normal. She's always lived in a bigger body and knew that weight loss wasn't going to "fix" her health problems. It never had, and the diagnosis didn't seem to be related to her weight—she'd never had health issues because of her size.

Jen's intuition told her to get a second opinion. Sure enough, her instinct was correct: She was diagnosed with bone marrow cancer by a second doctor. She asked if she could freeze her eggs so she could continue growing her family after chemotherapy treatment. This doctor was against it. Once again, Curran trusted her instincts, got a second opinion, and plans to grow her family after treatment.

If Curran hadn't advocated for herself, she would have died. Luckily, Curran is going through chemotherapy and is doing well so far.[1] Unfortunately, this isn't the case for everyone whose symptoms were written off as a "complication of being overweight." We live in a society where some people are more worried about gaining weight during a pandemic than actually contracting COVID-19.

Doctors and public health professionals alike shout from the rooftops that obesity is killing us all, that we must lose weight now before we kill ourselves. In fact, the word obesity is incredibly traumatizing for those living in bigger bodies; it marks their very existence in medical terms and as "diseased" regardless of whether the individual is healthy or not. For this reason, I will be using "o*y" to denote the word to give readers of all sizes peace of mind.

Still, no one seems to question the logic of doctors. Have you ever thought it was weird that the "O*y Epidemic" supposedly spread like wildfire in a generation that thrives on before-and-after transformation pictures, Apple Watch calorie-burn

---

[1]   Katie Kindelan and Jordena M. Ginsburg, "Woman Says She Was Told by Her Doctor to Lose Weight. Then She Discovered It Was Cancer," *Good Morning America*, August 16, 2019.

sharing, keto dieting, intermittent fasting, "clean eating," and getting in your "steps" for the day?

If we take a look at the numbers, the o*y epidemic really took off around the same time the National Institute of Health (NIH) changed the body mass index (BMI) scale and new fad diets, like the low-fat diet, became popular.[2] In the early 1990s, the diet and weight loss industry was worth $10 billion.[3] It's now worth over $72 billion.[4] In 1990, the average number of o*e people in the United States was around 12 percent, and according to the Centers for Disease Control and Prevention (CDC), that figure has risen to almost 40 percent since.[5]

Although those numbers seem stark and are often utilized to incite the masses to pull up their bootstraps and fight this deadly disease that's swept the nation (sarcasm intended), the o*y warriors won't tell you that the NIH pushed back the BMI scale in 1998.[2] That day, over twenty-five million Americans who were considered to be at a healthy, normal weight became overweight overnight, and people who were already considered overweight became o*e. Although the numbers seem to have skyrocketed over the past few decades, the increase can largely be attributed to manipulated statistics

---

2   Elizabeth Cohen and Anne McDermott, "Who's Fat? New Definition Adopted," *CNN*, June 17, 1998.

3   Thomas A. Wadden, Gary D. Foster, Kathleen Letizia, Albert Stunkard, "A Multicenter Evaluation of a Proprietary Weight Reduction Program for the Treatment of Marked Obesity," Deception and Fraud in the Diet Industry, Part IV Hearing 102 no. 78 (May 1992): 961.

4   John LaRosa, "Top 9 Things to Know About the Weight Loss Industry," *Market Research Blog*, March 6, 2019.

5   Centers for Disease Control and Prevention (CDC), "Obesity and Overweight," National Center for Health Statistics. Last Reviewed February 28, 2020.

and increased rates of dieting, which we'll talk about in more depth later.

Think about it. We've been told that we're the generation that's become too big. Did we really become big, or was this data changed due to the NIH's decision to push back the BMI scale? Why isn't it common knowledge that this happened in the '90s? Why weren't we taught that in health class?

Could the increase in pursuing weight loss be what's making us bigger?

As dieting and o*y fearmongering have increased, so has fatphobia. Fatphobia is the fear and dislike of fat people. It's the stigmatization of and discriminatory aversion to fat bodies that our society has developed that shames and excludes people in larger bodies. According to a study published in the *International Journal of O*y*, weight discrimination is as pervasive as race and gender discrimination and has increased by 66 percent in the last decade.[6] Reuters, a news agency, took a poll asking people what they blamed o*y on; over 60 percent believed that o*y was a result of "making personal choices about exercising and eating" when we know that socioeconomic status, trauma, medical history, medications, history of dieting, and genetics play a role in body size.[7]

Experiencing fatphobia also has negative mental health implications. Weight stigma is associated with anxiety, depression, disordered eating, and eating disorders (generally

---

[6] R. Puhl, T. Andreyeva, and K. Brownell, "Perceptions of Weight Discrimination: Prevalence and Comparison to Race and Gender Discrimination in America," *Int J Obes* 32, (2008): 992–1000.

speaking, in describing one's relationship with food on a spectrum, there are healthy relationships, disordered relationships (think chronic dieting), and full-blown disorders), decreased quality of life, low self-esteem, and psychological distress. And while fatphobia has increased, rates of eating disorders have doubled. Between 1999 and 2006, the percentage of children hospitalized for eating disorders has risen by 120 percent.[7]

Fat shaming someone to lose weight actually does the reverse, largely due to negative mental health consequences associated with experiencing discrimination. So why are we still prescribing weight loss as a line of treatment? It doesn't seem like our attempts to improve health by losing weight have worked. The majority of Americans believe that weight equates to health. Doctors and patients alike believe that dieting is the answer to many problems. Arthritis and pain? Weight loss. Polycystic ovary syndrome? Weight loss. Fatigue? Weight loss. The list goes on.

I don't believe that prescribing diets and weight loss is ethical, evidence-based care. I believe that each person deserves body agency—the permission to be empowered to listen to your own body and advocate for its needs. Everyone deserves space to be here, no matter what they look like, where they come from, or what size pants they wear. Stories like Jen Curran's shouldn't have to be run on *Good Morning America* to highlight how damaging fatphobia is in our medical space and society.

---

7   Sharon Begley, "Insight: America's hatred of fat hurts obesity fight," Health News: Reuters (article), May 11, 2012.

But Hannah, what about their health?

Hear me out: We can promote healthful behaviors without prescribing weight loss or masked diets. I'm all for promoting the consumption of fruits and veggies, moving our bodies more, getting adequate sleep, and drinking water. We can encourage those behaviors without weight loss being the end goal, or even a part of the conversation. Increasing healthful behaviors has better health outcomes than weight loss does long term.

I was compelled to spend the past few years researching fatphobia and dieting after spending time in three eating disorder treatment facilities from late 2017 to early 2018. I learned from expert doctors, dietitians, and psychologists about our bodies, how societal pressures interact with health, and the long-term implications of dieting and fatphobia. The fact that members of the program had to prepare themselves for the trauma that can accompany going to the doctor made me want to dive into this subject further and develop a solution to the pervasive problem that is fatphobia.

When I told my doctor about my eating disorder, I heard him comment to another provider outside: "I can't believe she has an eating disorder. She's muscular and voluptuous, I mean she's glowing!"

That kind of comment is exactly why I am writing this. It is 2020 and medical professionals still lack education on eating disorders, nutrition, and where body size fits in health. There are so many antiquated stereotypes and platitudes about size and health that science has shown just aren't accurate, but we still continue to go off of old systems. We rely on a body mass index scale that's been manipulated over time and wasn't even developed to measure health in the first place.

Doctors prescribe weight loss as if it's a cure all when it can actually make problems worse long-term and cause people's underlying diseases to go unnoticed until it's too late. People are avoiding the doctor in fear that they're just going to be shamed and told to lose weight. Even after getting out of treatment and having a laundry list of things about eating disorders on my chart, I still have to debate with nurses to not be weighed, or to not be given the packet of paper with my old weight and BMI in bold at the top.

What I deal with is nothing compared to what people in bigger bodies have to deal with. After researching fatphobia, the history of society's thinness ideal, listening to people's experiences, and studying the methods of medical practitioners who offer weight-inclusive care, I have developed a theory that this book will defend.

Weight does not equate to health. To assume that it does is fatphobic, not evidence-based, and harming to our society. By taking back our body agency, we can advocate for the weight inclusive evidence-based care we need and dismantle antiquated, fatphobic norms that are hurting millions of people.

This book is for anyone who struggles with weight stigma, is interested in the implications of weight stigma, or has a loved one who deals with it. This is for anyone who feels they aren't heard at the doctor's office or have struggled and yo-yoed on diets for years. This book is also a great resource for medical providers and medical students who want to offer compassionate, equal care to all of their patients.

We'll explore:

- Why diets don't work and why doctors aren't qualified to prescribe them
- How fatphobia is rooted in racism and colonialism
- How fatphobia is killing people
- How we can advocate for weight-inclusive care
- How some medical providers are already treating patients with weight-inclusive care

For providers: Weight is a controversial topic. We've all grown up in a world that obsesses over dieting, thinness, and all things "health." Try to keep an open mind. It's not necessarily our fault that we got here, but it is our responsibility to unlearn diet culture and give patients ethical, evidence-based care.

For the rest of us: We are all learning, and I hope that the following experiences, research, and stories can empower us to take action and advocate for adequate health care, sans diet and weight talk.

ACKNOWLEDGING
MY PRIVILEGE

———

My intent for this book is to raise the voices of people in marginalized bodies to show the world that fatphobia in healthcare is not just some body positivity issue—it's a human rights issue. People are being actively discriminated against and not getting vital diagnoses that could save their lives because they're fat. Our medical system has been complicit with the systematic oppression of fat bodies. Because of this, people aren't getting cancer diagnoses in time, people are being put through weight cycling, which causes more health problems long term, and people are avoiding seeking medical care out of fear that they won't be heard.

Yes, medical fatphobia has been acknowledged and talked about, but nothing has been done about it on a larger scale. Health at Every Size doctors, I thank you for your work, and I hope that more providers will follow suit and practice weight-inclusive care in the near future. Awareness is the first step, but action must be taken in order to effect change.

That being said, I acknowledge my own body privilege. I am a white, straight-sized woman, meaning that I can go into most clothing stores and find something that fits me, and I've also had access to adequate resources throughout my life. When I came to my doctor to tell him that I had an eating disorder and was going to treatment, he was shocked because I didn't fit the mold of what society says an eating disorder looks like, but he believed me, though that's not the case for many people in bigger bodies. My insurance covered most of the cost of treatment, likely because I had a diagnosis that fit the mold for eating disorder stereotypes, and there happened to be an advocate for eating disorders in my insurance group. Often times, weight can be a barrier in getting diagnoses that are considered "severe enough" to get coverage. A lot of people have a hard time getting insurance on board, and I saw a lot of people's insurance get cut randomly a few weeks into treatment.

In the case of eating disorders, most people who suffer from one, but live in a bigger body, don't even get a diagnosis, much less get access to treatment.

When I ask not to get weighed at the doctor, I get pushback half the time, but typically, nurses will understand.

People believe me when I say I have a medical issue. I don't get told that it's a weight problem, and I don't get prescribed weight loss regimens. That's a privilege.

That isn't the case for most of the people I've interviewed that you're about to meet.

I recognize that my stories pale in comparison to those who live in marginalized bodies. That's why this book isn't a memoir. By hearing the stories of people who've experienced the trauma that is medical fatphobia in this book and analyzing the research that conflicts with the current way our society treats people in bigger bodies, I hope that our medical system and our society can begin to question our antiquated practices and treat everyone equally, regardless of size or appearance.

INSPIRATION STORY

I was twenty-one years old, sitting in my pediatrician's office back home from college because I had to get blood work done before heading off to eating disorder treatment. The results of my blood work would determine whether I'd go to a partial hospitalization or residential hospitalization facility.

"Dr. Suffolk will be with you soon," the nurse said after she took my blood and vitals. *Great*, I thought.

I had been struggling with an eating disorder for the better part of the decade; it had only gotten more noticeable to me (and worse) in college. I had been going to therapy for three years and had been in an outpatient program for a few months leading up to this point. I was miserable and knew if I didn't get help while I could, I might not recover anytime soon, if at all. I was afraid I was going to die of cardiac arrest one day.

I brewed in frustration, thinking back on how my doctor had seen my weight yo-yo for years and never asked any questions regarding my eating behaviors. I missed my period for a year and a half at one point, and he didn't seem to be too worried about it.

"It's probably just because you exercise a lot; you're healthy! If you don't get it back in the next year, give me a call."

I was angry. Angry at a system that only sees eating disorders in the extremely emaciated. The same system that worries parents over their kids getting fat but doesn't seem to worry too much about kids' relationships with food. Well, here I am.

Dr. Jason, a tall, wiry man, waltzed in, reeking of designer cologne, "Hannah, my girl, it's so good to see you!"

"Good to see you!" I politely responded.

Dr. Jason said, "Look, these things happen. It's gonna be okay."

He caught up with my mom and stepped out of the room, but I heard him talking to another person in the hallway:

"I can't believe she has an eating disorder, she's so muscular and *voluptuous*! I mean, she's glowing, she looks great. I don't see it."

I was *furious* that admitting myself into treatment wasn't enough evidence that I had a problem. The fact that I'd come into a physical in high school weighing as much as I weighed in fifth grade one year, then gaining a significant amount of weight the next year, and so forth, wasn't enough. The fact that I had binged and purged three times after my partial hospitalization program (PHP) that day wasn't enough.

It was that moment when I wanted more than anything to find a way to educate doctors on the harm that their "war on obesity" causes for patients. I live in a privileged, straight-sized body and was experiencing belittling comments on my serious illness. The lack of education, proper systems of evaluating health, and the $70 billion diet industry is affecting people's diagnoses and health.

At least when I say I'm struggling, people accept it. If I was living in a bigger body, I'd be getting prescribed extreme diets, diets that would usually be grounds for diagnosing an eating disorder in someone with a thinner body. I know that my stories mean nothing in the grand scheme of what's going on in our healthcare system.

My experience with doctors pales in comparison to the stories that are shared in this book, which have been told by people who live in marginalized bodies.

Fat people don't get taken as seriously by doctors. They get told to lose weight and come back if their symptoms still persist. What's worse: fat patients are often times misdiagnosed due to doctors' own biases, and it may take multiple opinions, persistence, or questioning to get the right diagnosis.

Fatphobia runs rampant in our society, and that doesn't exclude the medical field.

The obesity epidemic began around the same time the CDC pushed back the BMI scale. If you were alive in the '90s, you may have been considered a "normal" weight one night, then woken up to be considered "overweight" the next.

So after hearing my childhood doctor scoff at the idea that I was sick and describe me as voluptuous, I decided I was going to take a stand. I met people in treatment in all sorts of body sizes and backgrounds, and the more I asked questions, the more I learned: Fatphobia and diet culture are harming people in the doctor's office. Body size discrimination is keeping people from getting the diagnoses and help they need, whether it be a rare illness, a common one, or a serious disease.

I really don't want to live in a world where my weight matters more than my behavioral health or my physical health. I especially don't want to live in one where people are seen as lesser for being fat.

I hope that this book offers a call to action in patients and in medical professionals to reevaluate how we're approaching health, how we're defining it, and how fatphobia is making people's health worse, and in some cases, killing them.

PART 1:

WHEN AND HOW DID SOCIETY BECOME SO FATPHOBIC?

CHAPTER 1

DIET CULTURE'S HEAVY HAND

———

Diet culture is hard to ignore. It's all over our social media, on invasive ads, and on explore pages. You see it on billboards, in commercials, in doctors' offices, and at restaurants. We are told that we need to watch our sugar because if we don't, we'll get diabetes. We're told that sitting is the new smoking (which is ridiculous). We are sold cellulite creams, fat burners, and workout programs ridden with empty promises. "Clean eating" movements have demonized processed foods without regard for the fact that for many families in lower socioeconomic statuses, that's the quickest, most affordable way to feed their children. Weight Watchers, now WW, rolled out Kurbo, a diet program for children, that has games for kids to rank foods as green, yellow, or red according to whether the food is a good food or a bad food. Does that sound healthy to you?

In this chapter, we'll cover:

- What exactly diet culture is and how it causes harm

- Firsthand stories of how diet culture has negatively impacted people's lives, inside and outside of the health-care system
- And, when diet culture took off as well as how we got here

DIET CULTURE:

(n) a system of beliefs that worships thinness and equates it to health and moral virtue.[8]

(n) a system of beliefs rooted in patriarchal and colonialist ideals.

(n) will make you feel lesser for your entire life if you allow it, will call you a failure for not beating biology, or will at least make you feel morally "bad" for eating designated "bad" foods.

(n) has seeped into the medical industry and is causing harm to patients. Medical providers are human, too, and can fall victim to quack diet advice. See: Dr. Oz.

(n) has shape-shifting qualities that allows it to change over time to suit the palette of society's current interests, such as wellness, which has recently made it extremely difficult to decipher real wellness from the fake. See: Weight Watchers rebranding to WW. The new buzzword "wellness" has also proved to be a new way for diet culture to sell diets and unhealthy exercise regimens as "healthful choices" that are really masked disordered, unsustainable behaviors.

Diet culture is present in homes, at schools, at your kid's sports activities, and at weekly work lunches. It makes us feel

---

[8]   Christy Harrison. "What Is Diet Culture?" *Christy Harrison*, August 10, 2018.

responsible for our body's size, despite the fact that our weight is largely determined by genetics and a host of other factors. It sends the message that in order to fit in, we must change X, Y, and Z about our bodies, our appearance, and our habits. Diet culture says that fatness has no place in society; it must be eradicated at all costs, or else you won't be deemed good enough to succeed, thrive, and even find love in the world.

I believe it's very helpful to look at how one person's view of dieting or losing weight as a result of diet culture's messaging can affect those around them. It's important to recognize diet culture in our personal lives and see how it not only affects those around us, but how it also affects healthcare and how our culture practices medicine. The following are a few stories of women who've experienced diet culture and fatphobia in their lives, inside and outside the healthcare system. Although all of these women have gotten clinical help, they are still struggling today and dealing with the battle of wanting to nourish themselves properly without dealing with the repercussions of living in a fatphobic society in a bigger body. It's the catch-22 of today: Be body positive, but don't take up too much space.

The overarching message we receive from our culture is this: "We want you to be healthy, but if that involves weight gain, maybe diet just a little bit, so you're more palatable to society."

We live in a world today where people in bigger bodies can't exist in peace without being constantly judged, given advice, discriminated against, and hated because of their bodies. We're all told by the media, by our primary care doctors, and by our loved ones that "it's just a matter of willpower" or "X diet worked for me, it'll work for you too." The reality is our bodies just aren't built to be manipulated.

We aren't born to hate our bodies; we learn to hate them through the messages we receive or hear from family, work, the media, and peers. This is diet culture through the eyes of N'kyla, Sarah, and Amita.

N'KYLA

It's important to point out before sharing N'kyla's story that parents do their best to raise their children; I'm not here to blame or attribute anything to any family or caregiver's behaviors. It is no one's fault that we were brought into a world that tells us we need to shrink ourselves to be worthy of acceptance. In a lot of ways, these diet-culture-rooted beliefs protected many of us throughout our lives, served as a coping skill, and helped us feel accepted. In that case, it makes sense to want to pass down lifelong skills that allowed us to cope and feel accepted to our children.

N'kyla, Jade, Anna, and I danced together for almost a decade when we were younger. N'kyla's mom "struggled" with her weight and went on several diets throughout N'kyla's childhood. She had gone through a few minor plastic surgery operations, only bought organic, natural food at times, and would hide sweets in the house.

As a result, N'kyla would take full advantage of having access to "banned" foods at her house when she'd come over to mine.

"Oh my gosh Mrs. Hanks you have regular jelly? This is so good!"

You'd think peanut butter and jelly sandwiches were a delicacy.

"My mom served fennel as our dinner last night. I was so hungry I raided our pantry after."

This wasn't unusual at her home. My mom made a point to buy N'kyla regular Smucker's jelly and would make sure we had cookies or some sort of treat when she'd come over. Anna, Jade, and I used to joke that N'kyla was always hungry and could always eat, because, well, she was. Her food preferences weren't satisfied at home, so she'd make up for that elsewhere. One time she bought a cake at the grocery store for a sleepover and ended up eating it all herself.

You might think that this sort of behavior isn't normal for a kid—and it isn't. Nobody was really concerned with her behaviors at the time; on the surface, there was nothing to worry about yet.

Until one summer, that is. N'kyla had to undergo an invasive jaw surgery that left her on a liquid-only diet for weeks. We didn't see her for almost two months, and when she came back to dance that fall, the difference in her appearance was stark.

"N'kyla, you're so skinny! Are you okay?" Anna exclaimed with concern.

"Oh, yeah. Because of my surgery I kind of had to live off smoothies for a while. It just happened!"

Anna was suspicious. "But you're eating now, right? You've never been a skinny person."

"Yeah, I am. My appetite has just changed some."

That was the end of the conversation. We thought something was off, but as fourteen- and fifteen-year-olds, we didn't know what else to say.

As N'kyla's disordered eating evolved and developed into something more serious, her body began to resist restriction. Her mother continued to encourage "healthy" eating and even suggested diets at times. One Christmas when N'kyla came home from college, her mom gave her some Weight Watchers pamphlets.

Fast forward a year. N'kyla realized that she had been dealing with bulimia and anorexia and sought out a therapist for help.

"I hid it from my parents because I wasn't sure how they'd react. My mom was so focused on looking a certain way that it was easier for me to tell them that I needed one therapist for anxiety and one for depression than to explain that I'd been struggling with this for years; they wouldn't get it and would minimize it."

Things didn't improve, and N'kyla eventually reached out to her parents to help her go to treatment. She's since had to set boundaries with family members to stop them from continually offering her diets and ways to lose weight.

SARAH

Sarah's first visit with a primary care doctor after spending a year in and out of eating disorder treatment was unfortunately not an unusual experience for patients in bigger bodies.

"Sarah, how are you doing?"

"I'm doing better. I just got out of treatment, as you probably saw on my chart. I'm still seeing a therapist and dietitian, which is helpful."

"Okay. What has your eating been looking like? Are you making sure to eat fruits and vegetables?"

"Yes, I've been following a meal plan that my dietitian developed for me."

"I see. Wouldn't it be great though if you lost some weight?"

"I just got out of treatment for bulimia, so we're trying to stabilize my weight right now. We're not trying to do anything with it."

Sarah's doctor started to look uncomfortable, but continued.

"Oh, well, you know, losing weight is still good for our health if we do it safely."

"Well, according to my medical history it's pretty much impossible for me do it safely, thank you."

"Well, you could still lose some weight. You can lose weight in a healthy way. You know, cutting sodas and sugary things, exercising more."

"I only drink water. I've been hospitalized for trying to lose weight."

"Oh, um, well, losing some pounds can still benefit your health."

Sarah fell silent and finished up the visit, receiving her discharge packet at checkout. Her doctor apparently wasn't convinced that Sarah shouldn't lose weight because of her eating disorder history.

"After talking to her about how I can't diet and how I'm seeing a dietitian and a therapist, the packet I was given not only had my weight and BMI, but it also had a six-page document that outlined how to eat healthy and exercise, and how losing ten pounds can benefit your health. I had just told her I recently got out of eating disorder treatment and am working with a dietitian."

"I was consumed with the eating disorder for so long, so, obviously, I've tried to lose weight. But it's impossible for me to do that in a healthy way, and we know now that the evidence says that going on diets and trying to lose weight doesn't work long term. My body is going to bounce back and I'm going to do more damage to my metabolism and probably end up gaining more weight and have to go back to treatment for an eating disorder. My chart says I've been hospitalized for this and that I've had to get a lot of help for it, so I felt like I wasn't heard. It honestly felt really belittling."

AMITA

Amita came from India to the United States to obtain a master's in business administration at the University of Minnesota. She was shocked and disheartened to learn that despite the US being the home of the body positive movement, people judged her and made comments to her about her body size. She started seeing a therapist for disordered eating, which has helped her cope, but she explains how it's hard to accept her body for the way it is in a world that doesn't want her to love herself.

"I've been a little bigger since I was six or seven. The way it is talked about here is very different. In India, people would say, 'yeah this person is fat,' make some remarks, and that's it. But here, it's like there's an assumption that this person doesn't take care of themselves, which I find a lot worse, because that's a judgment against who I am as a person. I've heard a lot of people talk about this like, they don't take time out for themselves or don't think of themselves as a priority.

"I've heard a lot of people say that 'I'm thin because I take care of my health,' which is a very passive way of saying if you're fat, you just don't take care of your health. And this connection with health is very interesting because I had never seen it before. [In India] being fat was considered bad, but it was just one thing; it was never considered a judgment against me. Here, I feel like sometimes when I enter a room, there's already a judgment made against me because of how I look."

Amita admits that it's hard to accept your body in a world that doesn't want you to: "I'll go to therapy and feel great and feel like I'm going to explore some of these techniques and then somebody will say, 'We just did this workout, why don't you start something like that?' Or somebody will say, 'Are you sure you want to eat out today, maybe I can make you a salad!'

And although they were delivered in a well-intended manner, they felt like micro-aggressions against my body. My body isn't meant to be small. I've tried to lose weight plenty of times, and it makes me feel like every time I enter a room there's a judgment made about me, that I'm lazy or don't take care of myself."

N'kyla, Sarah, and Amita all experienced some form of oppression through diet culture and internalized fatphobia in our society. Had N'kyla never been exposed to the idea that we can supposedly control our body size by controlling our food, she may have never developed an eating disorder. If Sam lived in a smaller body, her healthcare provider wouldn't have even mentioned weight and would likely have given her a pat on the back for seeking help for her eating disorder and ended the conversation there. Amita moved continents away from family to pursue further education and continues to deal with fatphobic, diet-culture-ridden comments from peers about her body. If she were thin, she wouldn't have to experience this and could probably focus on her studies better.

My friend's work office has weight loss challenges regularly, and right now the office has a water challenge. Whoever drinks the most water wins. She took me into her office one day during my lunch break to introduce me to some colleagues, and when one of them told me about the challenge, I had to hold my tongue. I drank too much water when I had an eating disorder and wanted to say, "You know, you can drink too much water. I've actually had to get tests done and go to physical therapy for it. Doctors told me I needed to cut back on my water intake because it's messed up my bladder," but I refrained.

Work lunch conversations are dominated by a colleague's gluten-free lifestyle or juice cleanse. Gyms and institutions offer cash prizes for whoever loses the most in "transformation" challenges. Every gym rat ran out and bought a thousand dollars' worth of gym equipment when gyms closed during the COVID-19 outbreak, and it felt like I couldn't get on Instagram or Facebook without seeing at least three home workouts hashtagged "no excuses." Some people have decided to take up intermittent fasting or Whole30 during the quarantine and feel the need to put it all over the internet. Memes and actual articles instill fear around the "quarantine fifteen," as if that's worse than dying from coronavirus. I used to not notice this stuff; if anything, I thought that the media, and the public, were simply promoting health.

But after going to eating disorder treatment and learning about the truth of weight loss and the diet industry, I can't unsee this stuff. It's everywhere. It's fatphobic. And it's harming people. It sends the message that being in a larger body is not okay, and it triggers people with histories of disordered eating. If you lived in a bigger body and saw a thinner person's transformation or saw a thinner person "fighting the quarantine fifteen" or the "freshman fifteen" in college or whatever is going on at the time, you would know that it feels terrible. People going to great lengths to not look like you is more than degrading; it implies that being in a bigger body is the worst possible outcome. Our culture confirms this idea, and unless we actively do something about it, it's not going to change any time soon.

We've been brainwashed to believe that if we eat a certain way, follow a certain diet perfectly, and find the perfect workout routine, we can shape our bodies however we want and be thin and healthy forever!

Fortunately (or unfortunately), it's just not that simple. Like Amita's friend who offered her a salad, she probably thought that she was being helpful, or considered the old "I care about her health!" argument. The truth is, this isn't about health. If we cared so much about health, we wouldn't be tormenting our fat friends with comments like "you shouldn't eat that" or "you know, if you could just start exercising more you could really shed some pounds."

Try to put yourself in the person receiving those comments' shoes. Does that feel good? Like someone cares for your health? Starving ourselves and forcing our bodies through workouts when we're tired isn't healthy. Denying our body of its wants and needs isn't healthy. Prescribing a fat person a diet that would be diagnosed as an eating disorder in a thin person sure isn't healthy either. But our society does it anyway—even though we've learned and proven that long-term weight loss isn't sustainable for about 95 percent of the population. Our beauty ideals and health measures have intertwined into one confusing mess that isn't evidence-based. Much of our medical system has co-opted our cultural ideals into treatment, but if we know dieting isn't sustainable, why do we continue to encourage it?

Diet culture tells us that if we can get our bodies to look a certain way, then we will be worthy of love, acceptance, that new job we want to apply for, etc., but what usually happens? We get to that weight, think we're going to finally feel happy or whatever it was we expected, and we don't. Maybe we feel better because we get treated better, but that lurking fear of gaining that weight back remains. And we eventually gain it back.

WHY DIETING DOESN'T WORK

How sure are we that we will gain it back? A study done at UCLA analyzed thirty-one long-term studies of dieting on tens of thousands of people and found that one of the biggest predictors of future weight gain was having lost weight on a diet at some point. But dieters don't only just gain back the weight they lost. One- to two-thirds of dieters gained more weight back than they lost within four to five years of losing weight.[9]

Psychologist Traci Mann, head of the Eating Lab at the University of Minnesota, has also studied dieters for over twenty years and reached the same conclusion. Mann says, "The evidence is clear. It couldn't be easier to see . . . Long-term weight loss happens to only the smallest minority of people," which is less than 5 percent.[10, 11]

As much as we're told to believe that we can control our body size, biology doesn't want us to. Humans have survived strife and famine, and we can thank evolution for that—our bodies work to keep weight on to survive. When it senses a famine,

---

[9] Stuart Wolpert, "Dieting Does Not Work, UCLA Researchers Report," *UCLA Newsroom: Science and Technology*, April 3, 2007.

[10] Kelly Crowe, "Obesity Research Confirms Long-Term Weight Loss Almost Impossible," *CBC News*, June 4, 2014.

[11] Roberto A. Ferdman, "Why Diets Don't Actually Work, According to a Researcher Who Has Studied Them for Decades," *Washington Post: Economic Policy*, May 4, 2015.

or in today's world, a diet of sorts, three things happen to keep us from losing too much weight.

Neurological changes happen first. When we aren't getting enough food, our brains become overly responsive to food. Our brains make us notice food more, make food look more appetizing, and increase its perceived reward value to push us to eat more. Our body thinks we're starving to death and encourages us to eat more to survive. The second change is hormonal. The hormone that make us feel full, leptin, decreases, while hunger hormones increase. So, while dieting, you're hungrier and less likely to feel full. The third change has to do with our metabolisms. The metabolism wants to use calories efficiently, and when we're in a deficit, it will adjust to living off of fewer calories by slowing down, which means that it will burn fewer calories than it used to, causing us to hold on to more fat. It's a survival mechanism that's allowed humans to survive famines and catastrophes over the past several centuries.

So if actively losing weight is the most consistent predictor of weight gain, why does our society continue to create new diets and promote weight loss as a healthful behavior? If we know that dieting doesn't work, why does it seem like a new diet or "lifestyle" change is created year after year? Why do our doctors recommend we lose weight?

There are a few answers.

1. Our obsession with thinness is still so ingrained in our society and in medical systems that it's hard to walk away from it, especially when doctors are being told that

o*y is killing us and that they must intervene and help people lose weight. Insurance companies offer incentives to doctors who track patients' weights. Big Pharma pushes diet pills. Weight loss makes money, and unless there's an overhaul in health care's belief systems and measurements of health, such as the BMI, antiquated paradigms will reign, and they'll continue to promote weight loss.

2. Medical professionals fear that if people know the truth, that dieting won't keep you thin, that people will "give up" and stop trying to eat healthy and exercise. Many doctors also feel it is a moral obligation to address weight in regard to health.

3. The diet industry makes loads of money. The industry is worth $72 billion dollars right now, and it's expected to keep growing. That's a considerable chunk of the GDP. For reference, the industry was worth $10 billion in 1990.

4. Although, yes, men are also definitely affected by diet culture and struggle with disordered eating and eating disorders, women are the primary target of diet trends. For centuries, the patriarchy has utilized impossible beauty ideals to distract women. We'll stay quiet and submissive if we're starving and wasting time trying to look a certain way. If we're wrapped up in shrinking our bodies, there's a good chance we won't be taking up space in C-suites, in government, and in high-dollar industries. In Naomi Wolf's work *The Beauty Myth*, she argues, "Dieting is the most potent political sedative in women's history; a quietly mad population is a tractable one."

Are you angry yet?

Many medical professionals and even more diet companies know that diets don't work long-term. Former Finance Director of Weight Watchers, Richard Samber, even admitted that diets fail. When asked how Weight Watchers was considered successful even though only 16 percent maintain their goal weight for five years, he responded, "It's successful because the other 84 percent have to come back and do it again. That's where our business comes from."[12]

Despite what you may have been told by your doctor, by your friend, or even by a loved one, diet culture is harmful. Although it may seem harmless to try out the latest trend, such as Noom, Whole30, or simply counting your macros or calories, about one in seven dieters will develop a full-blown eating disorder. This number may seem high, but 35 percent of regular dieters will progress into pathological dieting, and of those 35 percent, 20–25 percent will develop an eating disorder.[13]

Eating disorders, specifically anorexia subtypes, have the highest mortality rate of all psychiatric mental disorders, aside from opiate overdoses. Dieting *kills*.

Regardless of your motivation for going on a diet, the risks are high. You have a 35 percent chance of developing a disordered relationship with food, and if you happen to be in that 35 percent, you've got a one in four chance of progressing into a full-blown eating disorder. It seems like not many medical providers know how much permanent damage it causes.

---

[12]   Lucy Wallis, "Do Slimming Clubs Work?" *BBC News*, August 8, 2013.

[13]   Catherine M. Shisslak, PhD, Marjorie Crago, PhD, and Linda S. Estes, PhD, "The Spectrum of Eating Disturbances," *The International Journal of Eating Disorders* (November 1995).

There seems to be a huge gap in data and practice, right? If we've studied this stuff for years and have the evidence to prove that weight loss isn't sustainable, why are we still so hung up on weight loss being a cure-all for our health problems?

In short, ignorance, systematic oppression, and a multi-billion dollar industry that feeds off of our fear of fatness is why our culture continues to practice weight loss.

Our society refuses to accept bodies that don't fit the mold of what's conventionally attractive or acceptable. We're told that comments about our weight are for the sake of our health, when really, they're for the sake of making people more comfortable around us. If we're fat, we almost always have to be doing something to "change" that in order to be accepted for who we are. We're fed lies that we'll reach success and happiness if only we lose X pounds, but the results will almost always be fleeting, and we'll end up on the next diet or program and repeat the cycle over and over again. If you've been a chronic dieter, you know what I'm talking about.

O*y researchers aren't blind to the truth either. Tim Caulfield agrees that his o*y research colleagues "tiptoe around the truth." In an interview, he said, "You go to these meetings and you talk to researchers, you get a sense there is almost a political correctness around it, that we don't want this message to get out there."[14]

That's not to say that every healthcare professional in the country knows this truth and actively hides it. I'm sure plenty

---

14   Stuart Wolpert, ibid.

of medical professionals still believe that long-term weight loss is sustainable; after all, a small number of people can manage to keep weight off. However, any long-term research study will tell you that sustaining weight loss for at least three to five years is almost impossible.

These findings aren't new. In 1983, during the same time period that low-fat diets were all the rage and the Atkins diet was gaining traction, authors Geoffey Cannon and Hetty Einzig published the controversial but #1 bestselling book *Dieting Makes You Fat,* a breakthrough collection of research at the time that was dismissed by several medical professionals.

MINNESOTA STARVATION EXPERIMENT

Let's look at data taken from the infamous Minnesota Starvation Experiment, a study done in the 1940s that highlighted the psychological and physical effects of eating less for an extended period of time. During C12, or the twelve-week control period, men in the study walked about three miles a day and needed to eat 3,210 calories a day to maintain their weight. In the next periods, S12 and S24, they ate 1,570 calories per day. They became obsessed with food, and some of the subjects binge-ate and experienced intense self-loathing and guilt afterward. Subjects reported irritability, depression, increased hunger, and loss of interest in sex. By week twenty, all subjects reached a "weight loss plateau" and could not lose any more weight. Some subjects actually gained weight in the last month of starvation. In the restricted re-feeding period following the restriction period, subjects were assigned an increase in intake by 400, 800, 1,200, or 1,600 calories.

In the final period, subjects were given no restrictions and could eat as they please. The subjects gained all their weight back, and on average, gained 10 percent more than they originally weighed. The subjects suffered from hyperphagia, or excessive hunger, as a result of not eating enough for an extended period of time. Men who had never experienced body image issues felt poorly about their bodies and struggled with binging.[15]

If you've dieted before, you may relate to that feeling of being chronically hungry after restricting your intake for a period of time. Hyperphagia increases the likelihood of binging. You might call this overeating "falling off the proverbial wagon" of your diet, which typically results in feelings of guilt and remorse. You vow to yourself that you'll try again tomorrow, and so the cycle continues: On the wagon, binge, guilt, back on the wagon. Weight loss is then followed by weight regain, more guilt, more remorse, and more vows to stay "on track."

Except you won't stay on track because your body is going to fight you until it wins. Overeating is often a biological response to not getting enough food, and until you start eating enough for your body, you're going to keep binging, and you're going to continue to wonder why your diet isn't succeeding.

Diet experts might call this phenomenon a failure of willpower, when in reality, it's you versus biology, and biology

---

15   Abdul G. Dulloo, Jean Jacquet, and Jean-Pierre Montani, "How Dieting Makes Some Fatter: From a Perspective of Human Body Composition Autoregulation," *Proceedings of the Nutrition Society* 71, no. 3 (2012): 379–89.

wins 95 percent of the time. Compiled research has proven that we are as sure that weight regain will occur after intentional weight loss as we are that smoking causes cancer.[16]

Yet, our society and medical system continues to believe that weight loss is the answer to our problems. O*y has increased, so we must lose weight to avoid this, right? Not quite. As rates of dieting increase, so have o*y rates. There's a lot more to this puzzle than dieting, however. Certain medications, trauma, socioeconomic status, genetics, and weight cycling play a role in o*y, contrary to our society's belief that o*y is a "personal responsibility" issue.

Apparently though, it's not so odd that o*y has increased while dieting has increased. Almost half of Americans are trying to lose weight.[17] Most weight-loss studies that are used in the campaign against the "o*y epidemic" are short-sighted and often use data that only spans across a few months to a year. Studies performed over longer spans of time show that diets fail. In fact, within 3–5 years after dieting, one- to two-thirds of dieters gain even more weight than they initially lost, but the diet industry would never tell you that. Your medical provider probably won't, either.

HOW DOCTORS TREAT O*E PATIENTS

The majority of our medical industry is still convinced that weight loss is the answer and blames people's choices for o*y. Weight stigma causes more damage than anything, though.

---

16 E. D. Rothblum, "Slim Chance for Permanent Weight Loss," *Archives of Scientific Psychology*, 6, no.1 (2018): 63–69.

17 Jamie Ducharme, "About Half of Americans Say They're Trying to Lose Weight," *Time*, July 12, 2018.

In a survey of primary care physicians, over 50 percent have negative views on patients with bigger bodies.[18] Those doctors believe that o*e patients are less likely to take medical advice, properly take medications, or benefit from counseling. They have less respect for heavier patients and view them as lazy, non-compliant, and unattractive.

Doctors engage in fewer rapport-building activities with larger patients as well. They're less likely to engage in conversations that lead to an emotional connection, which not only makes their counsel less effective, but also can make patients feel as if they're not being treated or seen as a regular human being.

Providers may blame this on technical difficulties that make it hard to treat larger patients, such as equipment that's too small to perform proper testing and examinations. But instead of looking at those issues and thinking, "Hmm, looks like we may need to change the equipment," many providers will simply forgo testing or avoid certain examinations. Surveys have shown that providers spend less time with larger patients than they do with thinner patients.[19]

This pattern has caused millions of people to avoid seeking medical care. It's also caused providers to take longer to properly diagnose people in bigger bodies than their thinner counterparts, largely due to discrimination, oversight, and assumptions made on their bodies without proper testing.

---

[18] Mollie Durkin, "Doctor, Our Weight Bias Is Showing," *ACP Internist Conference Coverage*, February 2017.

[19] S. M. Fruh, J. Nadglowski, H. R. Hall, S. L. Davis, E. D. Crook, and K. Zlomke, "Obesity Stigma and Bias," *The Journal for Nurse Practitioners: JNP*, 12, no. 7 (2016), 425–432.

The medical system and our society are blaming people for poor health when the medical system isn't giving people in bigger bodies equal, compassionate care. How are providers supposed to support healthful behaviors when their judgment is clouded by negative views about people in bigger bodies and they recommend non-evidence-based treatment methods like restrictive dieting?

How can we promote health without hurting people? And how can we advocate for ourselves if we experience discrimination in the doctor's office?

We must abolish discrimination in healthcare, and we must advocate for ourselves if we want to be a part of the solution to this massive, growing problem. We must look past society's body size ideals in order to give and receive adequate healthcare.

CHAPTER 2

RACISM, FATPHOBIA, AND ITS IMPACT ON THE "O WORD" EPIDEMIC

——

Jackie, a thirteen-year-old budding adolescent, had the day off from school on Labor Day circa 2007 and spent the morning at home, half-watching TV with her mom, who was off of work and folding laundry. They were watching their favorite show, *Friends*, when the phone rang.

"It's the insurance company, I have to take this," Beth, Jackie's mom, sighed.

Jackie quietly listened to the phone call:

"Hello? Yes, this is she."

"Hi Beth, yes, we wanted to call you to ask about your diet and exercise habits. We noticed that you've gained weight and that your BMI indicates that you're overweight and almost obese."

Beth's shoulders and demeanor shifted and, noticeably ashamed and uncomfortable, she choked out: "I've eaten healthy my whole life, I take exercise classes every day, I *try*."

"Well, have you considered going on a diet? Do you eat fruits and vegetables?"

Beth: "Yes, I am a huge advocate for healthy eating. . . . I've dieted most of my adult life!"

"Well, it seems like you need to do something to change your habits. You're overweight."

Beth: "I have huge boobs; I'm not built small."

Jackie started to back away and let her mom finish the phone call. She couldn't believe that her mom was just interrogated on the phone like that. . . . Her mom was healthy and very sensitive about her weight.

Her dad, Phil, walked into the room. "Who was that, Beth?"

Beth broke down crying, "The insurance company wanted to ask me if I'd ever consider changing my eating habits because I should lose some weight, they don't know me at all!"

Phil responded, "Oh sweetie, I'm sorry. That's BS."

Jackie felt so much pain for her mom. *How could they treat her like this,* she thought. Her mom is the perfect picture of "healthy eating." She's yo-yoed a lot since having two kids, but she's always been an avid exerciser. Jackie remembers all the diets her mom had been on—South Beach, Weight Watchers, some doctor-supervised diet that involved eating bars and shakes, just to name a few. Some women just aren't meant to be a size 4, and her family was full of built, tall, busty women who had been college athletes and wore a size 10+.

If her mom worked out almost every day and ate healthy, why was she getting calls about her BMI being too high? Why did insurance companies *assume* she was unhealthy?

Doctors and other medical providers are shown piles of studies in school that *correlate* being obese with increased risk for diseases, such as diabetes and cardiovascular disease but aren't shown studies that prove that it is in fact weight, not other factors, that causes these issues. Med school or not, we're taught that thinness equals health, no ifs, ands, or buts, even though being underweight—not overweight—doubles your risk of dying.[20] Doctors are told in school that the BMI is the best way we can roughly measure whether someone is healthy or not without having to take out a measuring tape, or worse, run a lean body mass test.

What we don't take into account, however, is the fact that a. correlation does not equal causation, and b. the BMI system was created by a man who also co-founded positivist criminology—a form of eugenics that falsely determined whether someone was a criminal or not by physical features,

---

20 Alan Mozes, "Underweight Even Deadlier Than Overweight, Study Says," *WebMD*, last modified March 28, 2014.

specifically aimed at insisting that black people are inferior, savage, and criminal.[21]

Adolphe Quetelet, a Belgian academic who studied statistics, mathematics, astronomy, and sociology developed the Quetelet Index, now known as the BMI, when he was collecting data on "the average man," a social ideal meant to outline what a proper European man looks like. It's important to understand the context of his work: in the early nineteenth century, eugenics, a now recognized pseudoscience, was taking off. His index, which was based off of French and Scottish men, was eventually used to justify sterilization of people of color, people in poverty, people with disabilities, and immigrants.[22]

Quetelet had warned colleagues that his scale was not meant to determine health by doctors; his scale was only useful for his specific study. After all, taking someone's weight in kilograms and dividing it by their height in meters squared is an awfully non-holistic way of measuring health.

But when insurance companies grappled with self-reported, and often inaccurate, weight and height tables at the turn of the twentieth century in the US and couldn't figure out how to charge patients, the BMI seemed like a "good enough" fit for its needs. Back then, companies compiled sets of data for the purpose of having standard averages and "assessing risk" when taking new clients. However, the purpose of keeping

[21] Your Fat Friend, "The Bizarre and Racist History of the BMI," *Elemental Medium*, October 15, 2019.
[22] Alexandra Minna Stern, "That Time the United States Sterilized 60,000 of Its Citizens," *Huffington Post*, January 7, 2016.

track of these statistics developed into a methodology that the country could use to regulate its social norms and ideals.[23]

In the 1970s, researcher Ancel Keys tested the BMI's efficacy by studying seven thousand five hundred men from the US, Italy, Finland, Japan, and South Africa. The BMI could accurately diagnose obesity half of the time, but Keys noted that the index worked for "all but Bantu men." Once again, the system focused on white men, which raises the question of how accurate the BMI is for women and people of color.

Nevertheless, the BMI could diagnose obesity 50 percent of the time, which was better than the other two options studied: skin calipers and water displacement. Skin caliper tests involve instruments that clip onto your body to measure your lean body mass, and water displacement involves dipping you into a body of water. No thank you to both of those options.

Thus, the BMI was adopted by insurance companies and doctors alike.

The BMI's roots aren't the only racist aspect of our healthcare system's framework. We can't talk about fatphobia and weight bias without discussing its racist origins. I highly recommend reading Sabrina Strings' *Fearing the Black Body: The Racial Origins of Fat Phobia* to get a much more in-depth understanding of how racism spurred the United States' fear of fatness and obsession with thinness, and why it's still a

---

23   Amanda M. Czerniawski, "From Average to Ideal: The Evolution of the Height and Weight Table in the United States, 1836–1943," *Social Science History* 31, no. 2 (2007): 273–96.

part of our culture's systematic oppression of marginalized bodies today. This chapter is informed directly from her work, and I cannot thank her enough for the research she's done and the impact her book has had in this space. Again, this is not an exhaustive analysis of the history of fatphobia and racism; to get a thorough understanding, read Strings' work.

Two major events spurred the United States' fear of fatness: the transatlantic slave trade and the rise of Protestantism. During this period, Martin Luther called out aspects of the Catholic faith and started his own version of Christianity, and other (white) groups followed suit. Luther, among several other new Protestant leaders at the time called for justice for the people and moaned of the woes and corruption that were plaguing the Catholic faith at the time. The Catholic papacy held serious power in Europe, and the Protestants wanted that to change. The debate between which faith was the right faith eventually began a long, drawn out series of wars between Catholics and Protestants that really boiled down to power. The cry for justice during the rise of Protestantism was really a cry for justice for white people, and white people only.

Luther wrote up a list, *95 Theses*, that outlines his arguments against the Catholic faith. He wrote the *Five Solas*, which translated were: By Grace Alone, By Faith Alone, In Christ Alone, According to Scripture Alone, and lastly, For God's Glory Alone. These were circulated all over, and his faith took hold.[24]

---

[24] Marc Minter, "Luther & the 'Five Solas' of the Reformation," *Wordpress*, April 12, 2014; "The Five Solas," Introduction to Protestantism, Accessed April 2020.

Protestants were against the seeming gluttony and opulence of the Catholic faith. Much of that was applied to how they built churches, how they drank, and how they fed themselves. Rather than constructing beautiful basilicas, they believed in keeping the church building simple and conservative. In the same way, the sin of gluttony was very much intertwined in how they nourished themselves. Magazines and literature of the times focused on self-restraint in terms of indulgences including alcohol consumption, food consumption, and sexual behaviors.

As a result, upper-class Protestant women tempered their diets and grew thin to virtue-signal their devotion to God.

This was a change from the past ideals—being plump formerly suggested health, wealth, fertility, and beauty, but eventually this trait was seen as greedy and not in Christ's image.

While these new ideals sprouted up in literature and in churches across Europe and the United States, slavery and colonialism were still taking place. While Protestants were focused on bringing "justice" to people of faith, they were still faced with the dilemma of slavery: Was it ethical and aligned with their values?

This is where eugenics came into play.

Spiritual leaders at the time utilized religious guidelines to denigrate Africans. By painting a picture that Africans were gluttonous, overtly sexual, and lazy, not only could Europeans prop themselves up as the superior racial class, they could also deem Africans heathens who had no God and thus were lowly, unworthy peoples.

You see, fatphobia wasn't a byproduct of medical discoveries. Fatphobia was an intentionally crafted social construct that began during the Renaissance and came to fruition by the Enlightenment era. The concept insisted fatness was a sign of laziness, feeble-mindedness, "savagery," and racial inferiority. This false conviction was part of the scripted literature that laid the foundation for the eugenics movement in the twentieth century, which was used to justify the largest overtly racist regimes in the United States, Europe, and South Africa.

Developments of this idea began to spawn from European academics during the Enlightenment. Georges Buffon, for example, wrote a chapter titled "Of the Varieties in the Human Species" that argued physical differences between people of different races existed. He asserted that color, followed by body shape, were the most notable differences between races. At the time, it was believed that Africans were small, but he claimed that that idea was inaccurate. In his work, he wrote that Black Africans were "tall, plump . . . but simple and stupid."[25]

Buffon tied plumpness to laziness (see a trend here?), which was received well by British intellectuals. Not only did this idea comply with the pious teachings of Protestantism, it also gave them a pathetic and flimsy justification to enslave and exploit Black people. People like Buffon were elected into scientific societies whose opinions were respected and seen as fact. Buffon was elected into the Royal Society, a scientific society of Europe, founded by Robert Boyle, who was

---

[25] Sue Peabody, *There Are No Slaves in France* (Oxford Scholarship Online: October 2011).

considered a philosopher and scientist at the time, but to us, is a racist, misogynistic guy who studied and determined beauty ideals and weaponized race to divide people into social classes.

Buffon wasn't the only one who studied bodies to develop racial classes. Diderot, an atheist who spent time in prison for atheist literature, wrote about the propensity for gluttony among Africans and alluded to the seven deadly sins in his *Encyclopedia, or a Systematic Dictionary of the Sciences, Arts, and Crafts* despite his atheism.[26] Prospero Alpini, an Italian botanist, traveled to Egypt and wrote:

"Can one desire anything more shameful than an obesity acquired through the infamous vice of the flesh and of unchecked sensuality? . . . This vice is so widespread down there that one sees most women flopped down on the ground like fat sows."[27]

Samuel Purchas of England commented on his trip to Guinea in 1625:

"They have no knowledge of God. . . . They are greedie eaters, and no lesse drinkers, and very lecherous, and theevish, and much addicted to uncleanenesse: one man hath as many wives as hee is able to keepe and maintaine."[28]

---

[26] Sabrina Strings, Fearing the Black Body: The Racial Origins of Fat Phobia (New York: New York University Press, 2019), 82–89.

[27] Christopher Forth, "Fat, Desire and Disgust in the Colonial Imagination," *History Workshop Journal* 73, no. 1 (2012): 214.

[28] Samuel Purchas, *Hakluytus Posthumus or, Purchas His Pilgrimes: Contayning a History of the World in Sea Voyages and Lande Travells by Englishmen and Others.* Vol. 16, (Cambridge: Cambridge University Press, 2014).

These so-called philosophers and intellectuals used this kind of rhetoric to depict Black people as sinners who have no moral compass compared to the European Protestant moral code. By using some of the seven deadly sins, such as lust and gluttony, they justified enslavement. When doing so, however, they also associated gluttony and having a bigger body with being inferior, lazy, and irreligious. Our society today views fatness as a sign of laziness and inferiority as a direct result of this narrative.

Sabrina Strings wrote in her work that the thin aesthetic took off during what's called the "long eighteenth century," which was roughly from the time of the Glorious Revolution in 1688 to the Battle of Waterloo in 1815. At this point, England had already brought back sugar and coffee and had enjoyed it for almost a century from its imperialist pursuits, and to its despair, saw its citizens get fatter and fatter. Social elites feared this unintended consequence and began to rewrite society's moral code to reel in their "refined" society. The "standards of taste" outlined by this newly promoted appetite restraint determined the standards of etiquette for how men and women should carry themselves, eat and drink, and become "beautiful" according to this shifting view of propriety. It wasn't enough to be beautiful at this time, and deciding what constituted beauty was left to the intellectual man, who was ordained the arbiter of taste. Men were in charge of dictating beauty standards.

It's not an accident that eating and drinking less became a part of England's "standards of taste." Fear of being like the racial "other" caused women to shrink themselves. Being thin at this time illustrated a sense of morality, piousness, discipline, and taste. God forbid any English woman be associated with the "gluttony" and "barbarousness" of an African woman, right?

Thomas Muffet, a Puritan reformer, wrote a four-hundred-page manual on how to eat and deprive yourself of food. Similar to a modern diet book, *Health's Improvement, or Rules Comprizing and Discovering the Nature, Method and Manner of Preparing All Sorts of Foods Used in This Nation* mourned of the stories of the uncouth, excessive Roman empire, and grumbled over the fate of the English nation, as he claimed the country was "making graves with their own teeth." Muffet even quoted Greek theorist Heraclitus, who touted that "the wisest Soul dwelleth in the most empty Body."[29]

To me, that sounds like some pro-anorexia content you might find deep in the bowels of Tumblr that may or may not get banned from the internet, but at the time, depriving yourself was considered a sign of real faith and moral restraint.

This type of literature became widespread, especially as questions were raised regarding the ethicality of enslaving peoples. In the 1830s, *Godey's Lady's Book*, a magazine aimed at women, published an article on femininity, race, and overeating. The article warns white women about looking like African women: "Some parts of Africa no lady can

---

[29] Moffet, Thomas, Christopher Bennet, and Thomas Osborne, *Health's Improvement, or, Rules Comprizing and Discovering the Nature, Method and Manner of Preparing All Sorts of Foods Used in This Nation* [...] corrected and enlarged by Christopher Bennet . . . to which is now prefix'd A Short view of the Author's Life and Writings, by Mr. Oldys, And an introduction, by R. James, M.D. (London: Printed for T. Osborne, in Gray's Inn, 1746).

be charming under twenty-one stone," which is about three hundred pounds, wrote author Leigh Hunt.[30] Hunt cautions readers that eating in excess will result in having a body that is not appealing or fit for a cultivated woman.

So while white women did everything they could to shrink themselves, John Harvey Kellogg, a racist, yet religious man of many questionable trades, argued the opposite. The invention of Corn Flakes was largely a result of his fear that white women were becoming too frail to create strong offspring for the white race. Yikes.

Kellogg saw the thin movement as a concern for the white population. He believed that women needed fuller figures in order to maintain the "superior" white race.[31] He didn't just make cereal—he was a doctor, a pastor, and a eugenicist who believed that eating a better diet would serve God, ease disease, and furthermore ensure that the white race kept its place as the superior race.[32]

Eugenics is a pseudoscience that was harnessed by white supremacist individuals who claimed it was the science of improving a human population by controlling breeding to increase desirable characteristics in offspring. This "science" is what propelled the United States into the Jim Crow Era, inspired Adolf Hitler to kill millions of innocent people, and influenced Apartheid in South Africa. The premise of every overtly racist regime in the world relied on eugenics to argue

---

[30] Leigh Hunt, "Chapter on Female Features," *Godey's Lady's Book*, April 1836.

[31] Kellogg, Ladies' Guide in Health and Disease. p. 169.

[32] Wilson, Dr. John Harvey Kellogg, 214.

its regime. Eugenics was and remains a way for white men to justify racism and the exploitation of the racial "other." The book *Racism* by George M. Fredrickson goes into more detail on how eugenics led to the three largest overtly racist regimes in history.

Eating too much went against God, but Kellogg thought that women were not eating enough. They must eat more of healthier foods, he said, but ensure that they aren't eating in excess. Kellogg feared that the mainstream woman's pursuit of thinness was the cause of increased infertility at the time, which made him worry that "inferior" races would soon take over the majority of the population.

As much as he has a valid point that being underweight increases the chances of being infertile, you can clearly see how problematic his rhetoric was. He also advised against white people having children with Black people because he believed that the Black population would go extinct soon because they had "bad blood."[33]

By the 1900s, the need for health insurance took hold, and thus the Metropolitan Life tables were created. The numbers from these tables were developed by looking at the averages of height, age, and weight by people who were already insured, who, you guessed it, were mostly white men. The tables read that being overweight at a younger age was healthy, but being overweight at an older age indicated that you should lose some weight.[34]

---

[33] Kellogg, Ladies' Guide in Health and Disease, 392.
[34] Brumberg, Fasting Girls, 231.

Although many doctors at the time spoke out about the dangers of thinness, more and more articles against ob*y began to surface, and while some argued that being underweight was a serious problem, others took the opposite position. O*y began to be considered a disease and was seen as the direct cause of other diseases. Soon after Kellogg's warnings of thinness and infertility, articles surfaced of o*y causing infertility. Dr. John Gaff wrote that o*y was the only cause of infertility.[35]

It may seem that these contradictory arguments were a result of undeveloped science at the time, but this level of contrasting beliefs still holds today in the land of nutrition and weight. You can find just as many articles on how carbs are necessary as you can on how "dangerous" they are to your health. Look at how diet culture has shifted from naming diets outright—most diets are now veiled as lifestyle changes, wellness programs, or self-care. I've seen countless influencers contradict themselves by saying they intuitively eat but also track their macros or say that they help clients heal their relationship with food, while also building the "dream body." Diet culture can be so confusing that it's hard to find the truth, which is exactly the point of it all: If people don't know what's best for them, they'll "follow the leader" more easily.

The medical industry wanted to manage women's weights in order to ensure the white race could remain strong. They first thought women were too thin, then they thought they

---

[35] John V. Gaff, "Obesity as a Cause of Sterility," *Journal of the American Medical Association* 28, no. 4 (Jan. 23, 1897): 166–68.

were too fat, despite the fact that women's average weights hadn't changed over time. Physicians' emphasis on policing women's bodies for the sake of motherhood remained a prominent focus throughout the late nineteenth and twentieth centuries, all in the name of racial superiority.

By 1985, the Metlife standard weight tables were overshadowed by the BMI and soon became obsolete. The BMI was comparable to the old tables, so the medical field quickly replaced them. Ironically enough, the samples used to develop the BMI were also largely white men, which makes it a more-than-questionable tool to use on women and people of various ethnicities. As many doctors today agree, the BMI is arbitrary and doesn't really measure health at all, yet it's still a vital component of clinical exams and insurance filing. You'd think that a standard index would stay the same, but the BMI has changed its categories back and forth since 1985.

It wasn't until the 1980s that the medical field paid attention to health disparities among minority groups in the United States. In Katherine Flegal's study, "Prevalence and Trends in Obesity among US Adults," Latin Americans were singled out as a population with increasing BMIs, but Black women were front and center with having the highest BMIs.[36] Black women with higher BMIs had lower rates of mortality than higher BMI counterparts, though. Rather than developing public policy that could bridge the health gap, initiatives focused on personal responsibility and named eating in excess as the prime contributor to o*y.

---

[36] Flegal et al., "Prevalence and Trends in Obesity among U.S. Adults."

It's awfully obtuse to blame caloric intake as the sole reason for o*y, especially given the times. Genetics play a key role in our body's shape, as well as seasons of life, stress, trauma, and social determinants of health. The "personal responsibility" argument plagues much of the United States as it's also Big Pharma's winning argument in the courtrooms when rolling out new opioids. You can see how problematic the personal responsibility argument is. It acts as if we all live in a vacuum with the same controlled variables. Personal responsibility is an elitist belief that disregards barriers to resources, healthcare, self-care habits, and life stressors. If every person in the country ate the same exact amount of food and exercised the same amount every day, we'd still all be different shapes and sizes.

Our society continues to demonize the Black body today in its campaign against o*y. News headlines depict Black women being measured by thin, white doctors, and medical professionals reprimand our society's eating habits and lack of activity as the cause for fatness. When one study surfaces claiming that o*y causes increased mortality, another study that analyzes more people for longer periods of time finds that mild or moderate o*y actually lowered the risk of death.[37] Regardless, the impact of fatphobia on the Black community cannot be ignored in medicine. Fatphobia, combined with racial discrimination, barriers to accessing

---

[37] Katherine M. Flegal, Brian K. Kit, Heather Orpana, and Barry I. Graubard, "Association of All-Cause Mortality with Overweight and Obesity Using Standard Body Mass Index Categories: A Systematic Review and Meta-Analysis," *Journal of the American Medical* Association 309, no. 1 (2012): 71–82.

health care, and the psychological trauma of living in an oppressive society as a Black person continues to hinder the community from receiving health care equal to that of white people.

Today,

- Black mothers are 243 percent more likely to die from pregnancy or childbirth-related complications than white mothers.
- Black infants are more than 250 percent more likely to die before their first birthdays compared to white children.[38]
- Even though Black women are less likely to develop breast cancer, they're 40 percent more likely to die from it.
- Black women are 22 percent more likely to die from heart disease than white women.
- Black women are 71 percent more likely to die from cervical cancer than white women.
- Black men and women are 20 percent more likely to report psychological distress and 50 percent less likely to receive mental health treatment.
- Black men have twice the risk of first time stroke
- Black men and women are 30 percent and 60 percent more likely to have high blood pressure, respectively.[39]
- Black men and women have a lower life expectancy than white men and women.

---

38 Joyce Frieden, "Action Needed to Cut Disparities in Black Maternal, Child Mortality," Medpage Today, December 12, 2018.
39 Cigna, "Health Disparities: African-American or Black Population," Last Modified April 2016

- Black patients are 22 percent less likely to receive pain medication and 29 percent less likely to receive opioids for pain treatment, compared to white patients.[40]

In a study that quizzed two hundred white medical students and residents on biological differences among white people and Black people, students were asked if certain statements were true or false. With statements such as "Black people's skin is thicker than white people's," or "Black people's nerve endings are less sensitive than white people's," 73 percent endorsed at least one false belief in the quiz. Regardless of whether a person in the sample rated high or low in false beliefs on race, across the board, students and residents rated Black people's pain as lower than that of white people's, suggesting that the sample believed the Black body is stronger and more resistant to pain.[41] Consequently, Black people are overall under-treated for pain in health care.

Black girls are 50 percent more likely to have bulimia than white girls, and the onset of anorexia occurs earlier in Black girls than it does in white girls, yet many don't receive treatment.[42] Doctors fail to recognize eating disorders in patients

[40] Salimah H. Meghani, PhD, MBE, Eeeseung Byun, PhD(c), Rollin M. Gallagher, MD, MPH, "Time to Take Stock: A Meta-Analysis and Systematic Review of Analgesic Treatment Disparities for Pain in the United States," *Pain Medicine*, 13, no. 2, (February 2012): 150–174.

[41] Kelly M. Hoffman, Sophie Trawalter, Jordan R. Axt, and M. Norman Oliver, "Racial Bias in Pain Assessment and Treatment Recommendations, and False Beliefs about Biological Differences between Blacks and Whites," *PNAS* 113, no. 16 (April 19, 2016): 4296–4301; first published April 4, 2016.

[42] University of Southern California, "Black Girls Are 50 Percent More Likely to Be Bulimic Than White Girls," *ScienceDaily*, accessed October 22, 2020.

that aren't visibly underweight, and because of racial bias and stereotypes, some doctors don't expect Black women to have eating disorders. As someone who went to three different eating disorder treatment centers in different parts of the country, I can attest to the lack of representation: In the three centers where I was treated, there was only one Black woman in treatment with me. Kiera shared in group sessions that her eating disorder was invalidated in the past because of her body size and spoke about how difficult it was to reconcile living in a bigger body that's not accepted in today's society, and having to actively choose recovery over trying to shrink it. Although the media portrays eating disorders as an issue of the privileged white upper class, Black women are as likely to report binge eating or vomiting as white women. Adverse childhood events, trauma, chronic stress, and food insecurity are all associated with eating disorder development, among other mental health problems, issues that public health initiatives fail to take into account.[43] Instead, you'll find articles on why o*y is prevalent in low-income communities. Our society automatically goes to the personal responsibility argument and blames fast food, "poor habits," substance abuse, and inactivity, when so much more is involved.

These examples only scratch the surface of how much discrimination Black people face in health care today. Racism and fatphobia keeps people from being properly diagnosed and treated in a health care system whose measurements of health were designed for white men. Fatphobia was created to oppress

---

43 June M. Tester, Tess C.Lang, and Barbara A.Laraia, "Disordered Eating Behaviours and Food Insecurity: A Qualitative Study about Children with Obesity in Low-Income Households," Obesity Research & Clinical Practice, 10, no. 5 (September–October 2016): 544–552.

people, and it's still doing just that, hundreds of years later. If you're straight-sized and complain of having shortness of breath, you'll have tests run on you to see if there's an underlying condition that needs to be addressed. If you're fat, you'll get told to exercise more and lose weight. See the problem?

If we don't actively work to dismantle the narrative that fat is inferior and something that must be changed, we contribute to systemic racism in health care and society. The social constructs that emerged during the transatlantic slave trade and the rise of Protestantism were meant to distinguish the upper white class from the racial "other," and did so by contending that Black people's "excessive eating" went against Protestant teachings of temperance and self-denial, thus making them less pious and inferior to the Protestant whites.

When we see today that fat people are often automatically considered lazy, unkempt, less educated, and overall less than, those assumptions come from the social constructions made up by eugenicists who sought to justify enslavement and racial superiority hundreds of years ago. It's still here today. It's still marginalizing people. And it's still reinforced in medicine. By defending weight loss, you comply with the white supremacist fabrications of the past. If you have in that past, that's okay—you are welcome here.

It's time to unlearn the racist frameworks we've been born into and break down the barriers of health care for people in bigger bodies. As a medical provider, it's your job to give the best health care to everyone, and as a human living in this world with privilege, it's your job to uplift marginalized voices and fight for equality. The work has only just begun.

CHAPTER 3

WHY WEIGHT LOSS ISN'T SUSTAINABLE: BIGGEST LOSER STUDY

If you've dieted or attempted to lose weight in the past and regained the weight back, you're not alone. You're also not alone if you work in the medical field and have had weight loss methods drilled into your head throughout your education as the first line of treatment for ob*y. In this chapter, we'll look at why restriction and intense exercise regimens don't work long-term by peering through the lens of contestants who lost massive amounts of weight competing in the reality TV show *The Biggest Loser*.

We'll look at:

- Why can't people keep the weight off once they've lost it?

And consider:

- Why do we continue to prescribe restrictive diets and/or intensive exercise programs to help people lose weight when we've seen in numerous studies that they'll gain it back?

In January of 2020, NBC's show *The Biggest Loser* returned for its eighteenth season after four years of being off air. If you're not familiar with the show, picture a group of fat contestants being barked at by lean, mean, and brunette TV personality and trainer, Jillian Michaels. Contestants exercise for four to eight hours a day and consume fewer than one thousand calories a day, which is less than half of the recommended daily value. On the show, trainers tease and push contestants with fearmongering comments like "You're going to die before your children grow up" or send texts saying "We've picked out your fat-person coffin."[44] The point of the show is to help very fat people lose weight quickly in the name of health, but is the weight loss helpful and *healthful* long term?

Numerous follow-up studies of past contestants do not say so. The *New York Times* conducted an interview of past contestants whose metabolic rates and weight changes were measured in one study years after they went on the show.

Let's take a look at what happened to contestants' bodies years after losing weight on the show:

Danny Cahill, winner of Biggest Losers' eighth season, lost 239 pounds during the show but has gained over 100 pounds back since he left. He noted, "All my friends were drinking

---

44   Maureen Callahan, "The Brutal Secrets Behind 'The Biggest Loser,'" *New York Post: Entertainment*, January 18, 2015.

beer and not gaining massive amounts of weight," Cahill said. "The moment I started drinking beer, there goes another twenty pounds. I said, 'This is not right. Something is wrong with my body.'"

After reviewing his metabolic rate testing, Cahill found that his metabolism now burns 800 fewer calories in a day than it did before going on the show. Cahill said that seeing that his metabolism was damaged allowed the "shame that was on [his] shoulders" to be lifted.

Cahill is no exception to this.

Dr. Michael Rosenbaum, a Columbia University obesity researcher, notes, "The difficulty in keeping weight off reflects biology, not a pathological lack of willpower." It wasn't that Cahill didn't have the self-control or discipline necessary to keep the weight off; his body was fighting back during a perceived famine, or in Cahill's case, a restrictive diet.[45]

Biologically speaking, humans are mammals; our organs and genes are designed to help us survive. When Dr. Rosenbaum refers to biology as the thing that keeps us from keeping weight off, he means that our bodies' systems do everything in their power to keep us alive. When food is scarce, our bodies recognize that and slow down to preserve energy. What does that look like? The body drops in temperature, the metabolism slows, digestion slows, the heart rate drops while the organ shrinks, and lungs, ovaries, and testes shrink.

---

[45]   Gina Kolata, "After 'The Biggest Loser,' Their Bodies Fought to Regain Weight," *New York Times*, May 2, 2016.

If starvation lasts long enough, the body will shut down, leading to death, but in the meantime, these are some of the things our body does to help us live through a famine. Damage from starvation can be irreversible and slow metabolism down permanently in response to a lack of food. Our bodies are intelligent! However, our bodies are not smart enough to recognize that our diet isn't a famine.[46]

Erin Fothergill et. al published a follow-up study in 2016 on fourteen *Biggest Loser* contestants to measure body composition and resting metabolic rate (RMR). Of the fourteen contestants studied, thirteen had gained back at least some, if not all plus more, of the weight they had lost. In the contestants studied, RMR was 2,607 ± 649 kcal/day before the show, decreased to 1,996 ± 358 at the end of the thirty-week competition, and after six years, had fallen to a mean 1,903 ± 466 kcal/day. In simpler terms, contestants' bodies burned significantly *fewer* calories per day than they did before the show.

In terms of metabolic adaptation, the metabolisms of contestants slowed to a mean −275 ± 207 kcal/day post-competition and had slowed to 499 ± 207 kcal/day six years later. Their metabolisms *did not bounce back* from restrictive dieting, which made it almost impossible to keep the weight off.[47]

---

[46] Susan Brink, "What Happens to the Body and Mind When Starvation Sets in?" *NPR*, January 20, 2016.

[47] E. Fothergill, J. Guo, L. Howard, J.C. Kerns, N.D. Knuth, R. Brychta, K.Y. Chen, M.C. Skarulis, M. Walter, P.J. Walter, and K.D. Hall, "Persistent Metabolic Adaptation 6 years after 'The Biggest Loser' competition," *Obesity*, 24 (2016): 1612–1619.

But contestants suffered more health consequences than solely metabolic damage. Kai Hibbard, a former contestant and now body acceptance advocate who published a book on her experience on the show, has been vocal on the physical and mental health consequences of the extreme weight-loss methods.

In an interview with the *New York Post*, Hibbard said that during the show, "My hair was falling out, my period stopped. I was only sleeping three hours a night."

Weight fluctuation stresses the body, causing hair follicles to become inactive.[48]

In the same way, a body that isn't getting enough food will not be able to nourish a growing fetus, thus the hormones that trigger ovulation stop being produced.[49]

To this day, Hibbard still suffers from hair loss and experiences irregular periods. In addition, she said, "My thyroid, which I never had problems with, is now crap."

If you're wondering why *The Biggest Loser* has yet to have a "reunion" episode with past contestants, you can probably guess why. Contestants can't keep the weight off because their bodies' metabolisms are permanently damaged from restriction.

Our bodies have been evolutionarily engineered to help us survive famines, so it would make logical sense why our

---

[48] "Is Sudden Weight Loss Causing Hair Loss?" *Business Standard: Health Medical Pharma*, updated April 23, 2018.

[49] "Stopped or Missed Periods," *NHS*, last reviewed August 2, 2019.

metabolisms slow when we diet. Our bodies are trying to preserve the little energy it's receiving. UCLA researchers Traci Mann and Janet Tomiyama found that people who engaged in weight loss programs gained more weight after two years than people who did not participate in weight loss programs. According to Tomiyama, in a study conducted over four years in nineteen thousand healthy older men, "one of the best predictors of weight gain over the four years was having lost weight on a diet at some point during the years before the study started."[50]

So if we *know* that dieters gain the weight back, plus more, why isn't that common knowledge, and why aren't we taught that at an early age? We'll continue to explore this mystery in the next several chapters.

---

[50] Stuart Wolpert, "Dieting Does Not Work, UCLA Researchers Report."

PART 2:

HOW FATPHOBIA IS MARGINALIZING PEOPLE AND HARMING SOCIETY

CHAPTER 4

FATPHOBIA AND HEALTH CARE AVOIDANCE

———

"I found another doctor for an annual checkup. At the appointment, he physically recoiled at the sight of me. He quickly told me I'd need to lose weight before I saw him next, then left the exam room. My body was never touched, never examined. I learned nothing new about my health and was left only with the searing shame of believing that even a professional couldn't bear to touch my body."[51]

This quote came from Your Fat Friend, the anonymous and incredibly powerful fat activist who has shared her personal experiences of fatphobia in articles for *Self*, *The Washington Post*, and *Elle*, to name a few publications. Unfortunately, she's not alone in her experience with medical providers.

---

[51] Your Fat Friend, "Weight Stigma Kept Me Out of Doctors' Offices for Almost a Decade," *Self*, June 26, 2018.

Fatphobia in health care keeps people from seeking medical care. Many experience this phenomenon, and the details of each doctor visit inform its negative impacts.

Sam lives with Ehlers-Danlos syndrome, a genetic disorder that affects connective tissue, skin, joints, and blood vessel walls, as well as other autoimmune disorders that run in her family, and has experienced many related health problems. Ehlers-Danlos causes joint hypermobility, chronic pain, chronic fatigue, headaches, and dysautonomia, a condition that causes dysfunctions in the autonomic nervous system that can severely impact automatic processes in the body, such as heartbeat, sweating, digestion, blood pressure, excretion, temperature regulation sensory sensitivities, and brain fog, to name a few. As a person in a bigger body, Sam's symptoms often get written off as problems that could be cured with weight loss, despite the fact that many of her symptoms can worsen from a lack of nutrition.

When Sam was in college, she had a flare-up of what was thought to be cyclical vomiting syndrome and was rushed to the ER, where she stayed for twelve days while doctors tried to figure out what was wrong. Normally, a patient in this state would be on a feeding tube, but Sam was not.

"I didn't get an ounce of food and was throwing up all the time. My doctor didn't even give me dextrose until I passed out from low blood sugar—all because I was overweight anyways."

She was not fed for twelve days under the care of medical providers.

Starving a patient is not only inhumane, but it can cause worse outcomes during illness. Our bodies need nutrition to heal and function properly—why would we deprive a population of nutrition solely because they're fat? According to hospital dietician Chantel Walker, this happens often to patients in bigger bodies.

Sadly, stigma causes many medical providers to believe that they must put patients on a diet while under their care, no matter how dangerous it may be. Doctors' negative attitudes toward fat people ultimately affect their level of care.

According to a study on attitudes toward o*y in nurses, the majority of participants believed that o*e people were slow, unattractive, liked food, and overate. Over half of the nurses in the study believed that o*e adults should be put on a diet while in the hospital.[52]

The theme that people who are fat "choose" to be fat runs rampant in our society, and medical providers are no exception to that. In a culture that fears fat as much as ours does, it's no surprise that people who work in health care do too. Often times, doctors, nurses, and even dietitians may believe that they are genuinely doing good in the world and helping others by taking egregious actions like not giving a sick person food for almost two weeks or making snide comments about someone's body—all in the name of health.

For those who've been bullied or have bullied:

---

[52] M.-Y. Poon and M. Tarrant, "Obesity: Attitudes of Undergraduate Student Nurses and Registered Nurses," *Journal of Clinical Nursing*, 18 (2009): 2355–2365.

Was bullying ever helpful for either party?

Did teasing positively impact your life?

Have shame and blame ever helped anyone out?

. . . I didn't think so.

Starving someone while they're in a dangerous condition isn't healthy, and psychological abuse sure isn't either. Yet some doctors still engage in weight bias in practice, and according to data, it doesn't look like medical school is changing those attitudes anytime soon:

A study that analyzed five thousand medical students from forty-nine schools found that 74 percent exhibited implicit weight bias, while 67 percent exhibited explicit weight bias.[53]

This means that a large portion of our health care professionals are weight-biased and treat patients accordingly.

I don't know about you, but that doesn't sound very ethical to me. Our friend Sam could have died from going without food while vomiting for twelve days straight in the hands of doctors. And I don't say that to be dramatic; when we don't eat enough, and especially when we vomit, our potassium levels deplete. If they drop too low, we can experience irregular heart rhythms, which can cause cardiac arrest.

---

[53] S.M. Phelan, J.F. Dovidio, R.M. Puhl, D.J. Burgess, D.B. Nelson, M.W. Yeazel, R. Hardeman, S. Perry, and M. Van Ryn, "Implicit and Explicit Weight Bias in a National Sample of 4,732 Medical Students: The medical student CHANGES Study," *Obesity*, 22 (2014): 1201–1208.

That might sound far-fetched, but it can, and does, happen. When I was in the grips of an eating disorder, I had a really bad night where I had used binge/purge behaviors and had to be rushed to the ER later that night with tachycardia, a condition where the heart beats irregularly and faster than one hundred times per minute, which greatly increases the risk of heart attack, stroke, or death. Luckily, I got medical help fast and was okay, but the situation could have been deadly, and the same thing could have happened to Sam, especially since one of her autoimmune disorders involves tachycardic episodes.

The doctor at that hospital put Sam at risk for experiencing this, all because he decided she could use a few days without food.

As mentioned earlier, Your Fat Friend has been through years of abuse at the doctor's office as well.

In one appointment, her nurse took her blood pressure four times because she couldn't believe that a fat person could have low blood pressure. She'd been told to lose weight as part of her treatment plan for issues as simple as minor infections to larger problems, like endocrine complications.

"Regardless of the condition that brought me to the office, the response to every question was the same: 'Just lose some weight. Cut out junk food. Drink more water.'"

Doctors never asked Your Fat Friend about her diet and exercise; instead, they assumed she was "doing it wrong." She would come into her appointments ready to discuss medical problems and her weight but would end up receiving a one-sided tangent on her need to take care of herself and lose weight.

"As if I hadn't spent a lifetime trying to escape my own skin. Every office visit left me feeling more and more invisible."

This urged Your Fat Friend to leave the medical space and take matters into her own hands, except this time, her quest to follow medical advice and lose weight developed into a very disordered relationship with food. She quit seeing doctors and began the descent down the isolated, yet societally praised, path of orthorexia. Orthorexia, not yet observed in the Diagnostic Statistical Manual-V for mental disorders, but recognized by eating disorder professionals, is a medical condition in which the sufferer systematically avoids specific foods in the belief that they are harmful and has an obsession with eating healthy foods:

"Controlling my diet became the single-minded focus of my quest for health, even as other aspects of my health declined. After all, if you're fat, weight is the only marker of health that seems to matter. I had learned that lesson too well."

Your Fat Friend tracked everything she consumed on apps and would ask servers at restaurants how much butter was used in making certain dishes or how many cups of veggies were used in a meal so she could track them.

The fear of not eating perfectly ran her life, but people around her saw it as a valiant effort to be healthy.

That's the thing with orthorexia; in a world filled with "clean eating" and "whole foods" dieting, people often see these efforts as commendable actions taken in the name of health and even self-love. Those people don't see what goes on behind closed doors:

Panic when you don't know the specific ingredients in your food.

Feeling like you need to cook everything yourself because you can't trust restaurants or other people's cooking.

Constant thoughts and obsessions as to what you'll be eating next, what you won't be eating next, if what you ate last was "good" enough.

Scrutinizing over MyFitnessPal and working diligently to meet your set macros (the slang term for counting protein, carbohydrates, fats) or calories perfectly, and if you don't hit them, the overwhelming feelings of shame and guilt that monopolize your headspace.

Skipping out on family meals out of fear that they'll "ruin" your macros.

Staying home instead of going out with friends so you don't mess up your food plan.

Finishing an entire bag of baby carrots because you didn't let yourself eat a brownie at your work event because of "sugar."

Your Fat Friend stayed away from the doctor for eight years.

Genny told me that it wasn't until she was sixty-seven that she began to have the courage to tell doctors she doesn't care to discuss weight and began to accept her body the way that it is.

"In my early thirties, I had moved back to St. Peters and my mom and sister had raved about a doctor they'd seen, and I needed a new primary care doc, so I went to have my annual with him.

Well, I came into his office afterwards and he closes the door and says, 'Well, I have to say you're morbidly obese. You know, your life is going nowhere. To be fat at your age is ridiculous, you know.'"

"At that point I began to water up and he interjected, 'That's not going to help you either.' The odd thing about the experience was that he was fat too. You'd think he'd have some empathy or level with me about my weight, but he didn't.

"At the time of this appointment, I was in the process of trying to get pregnant, so I asked him some questions about that. He quickly replied, 'Oh that's never going to happen. You're too fat for that.'

"He didn't run any tests on me at all. He went completely off assumptions, and this was my first time meeting him.

"I couldn't get out of there fast enough. I spent most of the rest of the day crying. In a private one-on-one setting like that where the other person has a level of authority over me,

I'm easily intimidated and can't stand up for myself. So after that I decided I wouldn't see a doctor for a long time, and I didn't. I was so devastated by what happened that I went years without seeing a doctor. Luckily, my health was fine, and I didn't have any health problems at the time, but I see now that stopping health care could have posed problems for me and put me at risk for letting undiagnosed issues worsen, had something been there."

At nineteen, Kenyetta Whitfield was excited to have her first gynecologist appointment. To her, it symbolized growing up and becoming a woman.

Those feelings didn't last long, though.

As she walked into the exam room, Kenyetta was quickly made aware that her body was too big for the exam gowns.

"This is the largest adult size we have," her nurse explained.

It barely covered her. "Why couldn't they have just given me a sheet that would cover me (like other doctors have done)?" she thought.

It didn't take long for the weight loss talk to surface at the appointment, despite the fact that Kenyetta's checkup indicated she was in perfect health.

"We'll have to work on you losing some weight," he said. "I can't let you remain this size."

Kenyetta's initial pride from taking care of her reproductive health fell as embarrassment and shame filled her heart:

"But that wasn't the first nor the last time a health-care professional would invalidate me. Later that same year my primary care physician suggested I lose weight to stop the insomnia I've faced for much of my life. The same doctor would also hint that my anxiety and depression were linked to my weight. She would then go on to suggest weight loss surgery while handing me a prescription of Zoloft to shut me up. . . .

"When you consider the instances of discrimination in health care that have been noted by both plus size and Black women, the intersection between sizeism and racism is obvious. How are fat Black women expected to trust health care professionals when doctors have demonstrated an inability to listen to our needs—the needs that will ultimately help keep us alive?

"The answer is: We don't. Instead, we continue to fear health care professionals and seek out medical advice through other avenues, or we suffer in silence. But we don't have to live in a world where medicine and medical care remain inaccessible to us. It is the job of health care providers to acknowledge and serve the needs of everyone."[54]

Black women aren't heard in today's medical field, and it's up to us to change that. Black women are three to four times more likely to die from childbirth than white women, and

---

[54] Kenyetta Whitfield, "Fat, Black Women's Bodies Are Under Attack. Why Did It Take a Thin White Man to Get Our Cries Heard?" *Rewire News*, October 12, 2018.

that's only scratching the surface of the inequities in health care they face.[55]

If we want to provide care for everyone, we must drop the weight loss talk from the conversation. In Kenyetta's case, there was no reason to bring up weight loss at her appointment. For many, facing these conversations at every appointment can lead to avoiding the doctor altogether. If you know what you're going to hear, no matter what health concerns you may have, you probably won't want to see a doctor.

Breaking down racism and centering Black women in the fight for equal care is crucial in eliminating fatphobia in the medical space.

Clearly, something needs to change within the medical system, and in order for that to happen, the work starts with us.

If you're not fat, you may find it hard to believe that this is what happens to people in bigger bodies on a regular basis. It's happening every day, and not only is it psychologically and physically harming, it's keeping people from seeking medical care.

In the past decade, weight discrimination has increased 66 percent, which is now comparable to rates of racial discrimination in the United States.[56]

---

[55] "Why Are Black Women at Such High Risk of Dying from Pregnancy Complications?" *America Heart Association News*, February 20, 2019.

[56] R.M. Puhl, C.A. Heuer, "Obesity Stigma: Important Considerations for Public Health," *Am J Public Health*, 100, no. 6 (2010): 1019–1028.

Yet, the vast majority of people don't challenge this kind of discrimination. Our society has so deeply ingrained in us that our weight is 100 percent up to us to control that people think it must be someone's fault for being fat. If keeping weight off was that easy, we wouldn't have a new diet or workout program coming out every month because it would have worked by now.

For whatever reason, our society thinks it's okay and even helpful to fat shame people "for the sake of their health."

Newsflash: Shaming and being downright cruel to people because of their appearance doesn't help anyone, and in the medical space, it's keeping people from accessing adequate, equal health care.

In a study that examined around three thousand fat women, 69 percent had experienced weight stigma by physicians, and women with higher BMIs were less likely to seek health care than thinner women were.

In the analysis, as BMI increases, so does experienced weight stigma, internalized shame, and consequently, health care avoidance. The higher the BMI a woman had, the less likely she was to seek medical attention due to previously experienced weight stigma that led to health care stress, body-related shame and guilt, and internalized weight stigma.[57]

So as the medical community aims to "attack this weight problem," they're driving away people who need healthcare

---

[57]   Mary Forhan, Ximena Ramos Salas, "Inequities in Healthcare: A Review of Bias and Discrimination in Obesity Treatment," *Canadian Journal of Diabetes* 37, no. 3 (June 2013): 205–209.

and causing some long-term collateral damage in the process. Weight stigma is a threat to public health as it affects individuals as well as the greater population, physically and psychologically.

Weight stigma in medical care disregards societal and environmental contributions to weight, increases health disparities among populations, and exacerbates social inequalities. Experiencing weight stigma has a reverse effect than it's intended to have: The psychological stress of being fat shamed actually contributes to weight retention, which makes it more difficult to lose weight. The increased shame and psychological stress around body size and weight discrimination can also lead to lower physical activity and increased appetite, which are caused by physiological mechanisms. Studies found that perceived discrimination, whether race- or weight-related, was associated with excess body fat accumulation. Weight discrimination has been found to be a significant risk factor for depression, low self-esteem, and body dissatisfaction.[58]

In another study that observed women with insurance and high access to health care who are considered o*e, 68 percent delayed seeking health care because of their weight, and 83 percent said that their weight was a barrier to getting appropriate healthcare. When the women were asked why they delayed seeking care, women reported "disrespectful treatment and negative attitudes from providers, embarrassment about being weighed, receiving unsolicited advice to lose weight, and also . . . that gowns, examination tables, and

---

[58] Y. Wu and D. Berry, "Impact of Weight Stigma on Physiological and Psychological Health Outcomes for Overweight and Obese Adults: A Systematic Review," *J Adv Nurs*, (2017): 1–13.

other medical equipment were too small to be functional for their body size." The percentage of women reporting these barriers increased with BMI.[59]

The point of health care is to improve health, not make things worse. If weight stigma is negatively affecting people's health and keeping people from seeking medical care, we're clearly not doing it right. In order to eradicate weight stigma, we have to educate medical providers on the harm that fat shaming causes and how we can promote healthful behaviors without focusing on weight loss as the goal. There's nothing wrong with encouraging movement and eating nutrient-dense foods without making it about weight loss. As we've seen in studies we've looked at earlier in this text, improving healthful behaviors without weight loss efforts resulted in sustained health improvements, while weight loss focused efforts did not.

We can't say that we're helping people's health by shaming and blaming people for their body size.

"But I care about their health" isn't true. If you treat them as less than, you don't really care about their health. If you're a medical provider or are just curious to see whether you're fatphobic or not, take Harvard's Implicit Weight Bias Test via https://implicit.harvard.edu/implicit/selectatest.html. This can be a helpful tool to assess your own fatphobia and work to identify changes you might need to make regarding your own thoughts and behaviors.[60]

---

[59] R.M. Puhl, ibid.
[60] Visit https://implicit.harvard.edu/implicit/selectatest.html. to take the implicit weight bias test.

It's no one's fault that our society is intensely afraid of fatness, but it is our responsibility to unlearn our society's messaging and work as allies and supports for people who've experienced fatphobia. Believe them, stand up for them, and have empathy. Nobody is perfect, but by working together to address our own fatphobia, we can help others receive equal care in health care settings and in daily life.

CHAPTER 5

FATPHOBIA
AND LATE DIAGNOSES

———

I was surfing the internet one afternoon between classes when I came across a story titled "My Sister's Cancer Might Have Been Diagnosed Sooner—If Doctors Could Have Seen beyond Her Weight."

Jan had visited her sister, Laura, the author of the article, one spring in California, down sixty pounds, visibly strained, and in pain.

At first glance, Laura congratulated Jan.

"You look great!"

". . . I wasn't trying," Jan replied.

Quickly, Laura realized something was wrong.

"Have you seen a doctor?" she asked.

Jan began to tear up and shared her story:

"My primary care physician had changed his practice into a concierge practice, and I couldn't afford to stay with him, so I saw an OB-GYN a friend recommended to me.

At the appointment, I explained my symptoms: vaginal bleeding, constant pelvic pain, and unexplained weight loss. The doctor didn't take my symptoms seriously, and rather than asking more, continued to perform a routine visit exam.

"He didn't do anything for me. . . . He just saw me as a fat, complaining, older woman."

Discouraged, Jan tried different elimination diets, cutting out dairy and gluten to deal with abdominal pain, all to no avail.

Laura encouraged Jan to seek counsel from another doctor, and months later, Jan finally got an appointment with her internist. A physician assistant examined her and accused her of trying to get an opioid fix for coming in with complaints of extreme pain. The physician assistant did take blood, however, and Jan received a phone call early the next morning from the internist.

"You need to go to the ER right now. The calcium levels in your blood are astronomically high."

An MRI scan revealed a large mass in her abdomen.

The gynecologic oncologist in the ICU removed a tumor the size of a volleyball, the largest he'd ever seen, from Jan that day. The cancer had spread from her pelvis to her bladder and lungs.

Jan went through several rounds of chemo treatment and passed that Christmas Eve, six months after receiving a too little, too late endometrial cancer diagnosis.[61]

This story struck me; was this an isolated incident, or has this sort of delayed diagnosis happened to other people with larger bodies?

I realized I'd seen a less extreme example of this in my own life. A friend had suffered from chronic pain and arthritis for years (arthritis runs in her family). She had seen just about every physical therapist in town and was determined to not have to depend on painkillers to handle the pain. One provider really emphasized eating well as part of her treatment and put her on an anti-inflammation diet. The provider assured her, "This will help with pain, and you will definitely lose weight, too."

Well, she didn't lose weight, and her pain didn't go away.

She started seeing a new doctor and found out that she didn't have sciatica; in addition to arthritis, she had a cyst the size of a tennis ball on her lower back. After its removal, and much relief, she scheduled a hip replacement.

"I thought that the anti-inflammation diet would help, but it was completely bogus. I didn't lose weight, and the fact that I

---

61 Laura Fraser, "My Sister's Cancer Might Have Been Diagnosed Sooner—If Doctors Could Have Seen beyond Her Weight," *Stat*, August 15, 2017.

suffered for so long to realize that really upsets me. I've been a healthy eater and exercised regularly all my life, and I'm just not meant to be any smaller."

As I continued to explore this topic, I realized I'd seen this in more places. *Stat News* wrote an article about Rebecca Hiles, who at age sixteen, started to have a persistent cough. Doctors chalked it up to acid reflex or bronchitis until seven years later, when an ER visit CT scan revealed cancer. Rebecca had her lung removed that year.[62] *Good Morning America* had covered a story about a woman who was also told to lose weight and ended up having bone marrow cancer. Jen Curran, a thirty-eight-year-old woman from Los Angeles whom we met earlier, experienced high levels of protein in her urine, along with high blood pressure during her second trimester, and was diagnosed with preeclampsia, which is a pregnancy complication often stigmatized as a more common issue among higher-weight women.

Jen said she "definitely put it out of [her] mind" and rested for the sake of her baby.

A few months after giving birth to her daughter, Rose, Curran's protein levels were higher than before, although her blood pressure was back to normal. The doctor told Curran to lose weight.

"It was like a slap across the face. . . . As someone who's been overweight on and off for most of my life, it hasn't been a health issue for me, but I didn't feel like I should argue with her."

---

[62] Jennifer Adaeze Okwerekwu, "In treating obese patients, too often doctors can't see past weight," *Stat*, June 3, 2016.

Curran couldn't speak up with that doctor, but she felt that something was wrong and needed to get a second opinion. Sure enough, Jen's intuition was right: She had bone marrow cancer. After the initial shock of hearing the news, Curran asked if she could freeze her eggs so she could continue growing her family after treatment. When the OB-GYN opposed this option, she found another doctor who supported it, and plans to continue her family once she's in remission.

Since being diagnosed with bone marrow cancer, Jen has begun chemotherapy and encourages others to be an advocate for their own health:

"Lose weight if you want to. But if you think something is seriously wrong with your body, and a doctor tells you weight loss is the key to fixing it, get a . . . second opinion," she tweeted.[63]

After doing some research, it turns out that these women aren't alone in their stories. In fact, people who experienced weight discrimination are at a much higher risk of death than those who have not.

According to a 2015 study conducted by Florida State University College of Medicine researchers Angelina R. Sutin and Antonio Terracciano, people who experience weight discrimination have an increased risk of dying. In a study examining eighteen thousand people from separate longitudinal studies, Sutin and colleagues compared people who had experienced weight discrimination and people who had

---

[63] Katie Kindelan and Jordena M. Ginsburg, "Woman Says She Was Told by Her Doctor to Lose Weight. Then She Discovered It Was Cancer," August 16, 2019.

not. People who had experienced weight discrimination had a 60 percent greater risk of dying than those who had not.

The following is an excerpt from the study:

"Results were consistent across both groups of study subjects. In both samples, the researchers accounted for BMI, subjective health, disease burden, depressive symptoms, smoking history, and physical activity as indicators of mortality risk, but the association with weight discrimination remained."

"What we found is that this isn't a case of people with a higher body-mass index (BMI) being at an increased risk of mortality—and they happen to also report being subjected to weight discrimination," said Sutin, assistant professor of behavioral sciences and social medicine at the medical school. "Independent of what their BMI actually is, weight discrimination is associated with increased risk of mortality."[64]

In another study done by Jeffrey M. Hunger and Brenda Major at the University of California at Santa Barbara, weight stigma mediated the association between BMI and self-reported health. In the study, BMI had a direct effect on physical health that became non-significant once stigma mediators were included in the model. Once weight stigma concerns and perceived discrimination were added into the model, they became significant.[65]

---

[64] Doug Carlson. "Weight Discrimination Linked to Increased Risk of Mortality," *Florida State University News*, October 15, 2015.

[65] Angela S Alberga, et al., "Weight Bias and Health Care Utilization: A Scoping Review," *Primary Health Care Research & Development* 20: no. 116, (July 2019).

What does that mean? That means that although at first, a higher BMI showed poorer health in the study, once weight stigma and perceived discrimination factors were accounted for, it was stigma, not weight, that was shown to negatively impact health.

In addition to the two studies conducted, women reported experiencing more weight discrimination than men.

It's important to add that it's no one person's fault that we grew up in a society that equates thinness with health. Idealized thinness has been ingrained in our heads through the media, through education, and through social aspects of our lives.

I used to be a personal trainer, fitness instructor, and "meal coach" and would put clients on ridiculous diets in the name of health, so you're not alone if you have, too. We are not perfect, and in our society, dieting and weight loss are often praised! However, it is our responsibility to unlearn our own biases and treat every body with the respect it deserves. We're all learning here.

CHAPTER 6

EMPLOYERS, INSURANCE COVERAGE, AND FATPHOBIA

Fatphobia isn't exclusive to the health care space; it's omnipresent and affects people in the workplace, in classrooms, in households, and in social groups. As we know, people in larger bodies have to deal with the stereotypes of being fat, such as being lazy, undisciplined, less successful, insecure, self-indulgent, and unattractive.

Because of this, fat people face barriers in the workforce. Some may think, "Oh, people need to get over themselves and grow thicker skin, it's not that serious," but fatphobia actually impacts hiring, pay, and promotions in the workplace. Federal Employment Equal Opportunity laws, or EEO laws, protect employees from discrimination based on race, color, national origin, religion, and sex, but they don't protect employees from fatphobia. Michigan is the only state that explicitly added weight discrimination protection into the law.[66] In 1960, Michigan held a constitutional convention where eleven women were elected as delegates. These women were the first and only women to participate in a state convention of this kind. Daisy Elliot, a Black woman, was at the forefront of this bipartisan bill and worked for almost a decade to get a republican signature on it. She went on to become a state representative and served in the Michigan House for almost twenty years. If it wasn't for her, this bill wouldn't have come into law.[67]

In a study published by *Science Direct*, 45 percent of employers were less inclined to recruit someone for hire if they were o*e.[68] A study from Yale that analyzed around two thousand five hundred individuals who were considered o*e found that they earned up to 6 percent less than their straight-sized coworkers. Individuals in the study were promoted less often and were less likely to be hired.

Twenty-seven percent of women in another study of almost three thousand people reported weight-based employment discrimination. In that study, 43 percent of "overweight" people had experienced weight bias from employees and supervisors.[69]

This clearly goes deeper than hurt feelings.

---

[66] Lesley Kinzel, "New Study Finds That Weight Discrimination in the Workplace is Just as Horrible and Depressing as Ever," *Time*, November 28, 2014.

[67] Stateside Staff, "The Political Pioneer Who Gave Michigan's Civil Rights Law Its Name," *Michigan Radio*, March 10, 2020.

[68] Rubina Ahmed-Haq, "Fatphobia in the Workplace Can Be Career Limiting and Psychologically Harmful," *CBC News*, November 1, 2018.

[69] Michael O'Neill, "Fatphobia: America's Overlooked Form of Discrimination," *Brown Political Review*, October 10, 2016.

A 2014 study found that women who are considered o*e are on average paid less than non-o*e women and were less likely to work public-facing jobs.[70] This study held true even when education levels were accounted for. The correlation between wages and men's weight, however, was insignificant. Fat women are paid less, while thin women are paid more. A study that analyzed women's body sizes and wages using the categories of "very thin," "thin," "average," "heavy," and "very heavy" discovered that the thinner women are, the more they earn in the workforce. While "very thin" women earned $22,000 more, "very heavy" women earned $19,000 less.[71] That is a startling disparity in pay for something that's so aesthetic-focused.

Not only do fat people face wage, hiring, and promotion disparities, they also face higher rates for health insurance coverage. Although the Affordable Care Act bans insurance providers from denying coverage or charging higher rates on people with pre-existing conditions, weight isn't a part of that ban. In other words, it's legal to charge higher rates or deny coverage based upon weight. Legally, insurance companies are allowed to charge people more based on BMI. People with a BMI above 30 can potentially see up to a 25 percent increase in insurance premiums, and people with a BMI above 39 can see a 50 percent higher rate than someone with a "normal" BMI of 25.[72]

---

[70] Jennifer Bennett Shinall, "Occupational Characteristics and the Obesity Wage Penalty," *Vanderbilt Law and Economics Research Paper* no. 16–12, *Vanderbilt Public Law Research Paper* no. 16–23, (October 7, 2015).

[71] Lesley Kinzel, ibid.

[72] Amy Fontinelle, "How Much Does Health Insurance Cost?" *Investopedia*, last updated Oct 28, 2019.

Employers can require "wellness programs" to assess employee's insurance premiums. Some of these programs empower managers to develop weight loss goals for coworkers, and if coworkers cannot meet them, they could face steeper insurance fees.

The programs that a number of insurance agencies have rolled out allow employers to charge employees extra for being overweight. Imagine being pressured to lose weight by your employer. Is that ethical? Is it ethical to charge someone more for insurance benefits because they weigh more?

In 2006, the Health Insurance Portability and Accountability Act (HIPPAA) established a regulation that allows employers to penalize employees and charge up to 20 percent more for the total cost of insurance, whether it be individual or a family health benefits coverage, if they miss a wellness target, such as not meeting set BMI guidelines or having high blood pressure. This increased to 30 percent in 2014 under the Affordable Care Act. So, everyone should have affordable health care, except fat people??

Imagine your employer suggests you start taking exercise classes or reach a weight goal as an alternative option to avoid the penalty in your monthly premium. If you don't meet those stakes, you're still going to accumulate a different financial penalty.

Sounds like a lose-lose situation, right?

In 2013, a report found that 16 percent of employers require "wellness" programs in order to access benefits. Almost 70 percent of them set weight goals, yet only 59 percent actually offer help to achieve weight loss (which we all know won't last long anyway). These programs typically don't cover o*y medication, weight loss surgery, or other o*y treatments, and patients have to fight to receive coverage for them.

Let me get this straight: Employers are allowed to make people pay more for health benefits because they don't fit into certain BMI categories, which we have learned are flawed and not an accurate measure of health at all, and this isn't considered discrimination? Insurance companies can charge you more for weighing more, yet don't always cover weight loss options?

Where is the outrage on this?

Legally, HIPPAA protects you from disclosing personal health information to outside parties, such as employers. The ADA makes it illegal to force employees to answer questions or participate in medical exams unless the questions directly impact job performance, which is a slippery slope to begin with. Yet, 3 percent of companies that employ two hundred or more people require staff to complete a health risk assessment in order to get health insurance benefits. CVS and Honeywell (which was sued by the EEOC for its "voluntary programs") are examples of companies that require these types of assessments.[73] How would you like your employer to have your personal responses to questions like:

"Are you happy in your marriage?"

---

[73] "The Surprisingly Personal Health Questions Your Employer Can Ask You," *Money*, November 19, 2014.

"Do you smoke?"

"How often do you drink?"

"How many times a week do you exercise?"[74]

I personally don't like to mix my personal life with my work life and would feel a huge intrusion of privacy if I was required to disclose personal health questions with my employer. It's inappropriate for a manager to know the state of someone's personal relationship, the length of their health conditions and history, or their exercise schedule. I highly doubt that people are going to answer these questions honestly anyway. Yet, if you decline to answer these questions when you have an employer who requires them, you are charged a fee.

Employers have the power and legality to ask personal information that's supposed to be protected by HIPPAA, and can set weight loss goals for you?

And if you don't meet those goals, you have to pay up?

Maybe you meet the goal and keep it off for a year or two, but as we've learned, weight loss isn't sustainable. You'll gain it back and get penalized again.

An anonymous person who wrote about their company's health care benefits program shared that if they didn't

---

[74]   Abby Ellin, "How Obamacare Allows Companies to Punish Fat Employees," *Observer*, September 16, 2015.

participate in the annual exam, they'd be dropped to the lowest level of health care coverage, but if they did take it and "failed" any of the categories that were tested, such as weight, blood work, or blood pressure, they'd have to talk to a "health counselor" or see a general practitioner to get a clearance letter.

Some of those options may sound reasonable, but it's not so reasonable when employees are pressed to meet short deadlines to complete these tests. Jumping through hoops to take time out of your workday to hope that your practitioner will clear you is less than ideal. And if you don't "pass" the tests in time, you're bumped to the lowest level of coverage, regardless of whichever level you chose initially.

What was worse, this person said, was that you could only pass the weight portion of the exam if your BMI was a 25 or lower. For reference, someone who is five foot eight inches tall and weighs 165 pounds barely cuts it, as they'd sit at a 25.1 BMI.

This person had gastric bypass surgery and lost over 200 pounds and still didn't meet the requirements to pass the exam. The insurance plan didn't cover o*y medications, gastric bypass aftercare, complications that may arise from it, labs, or the cost of other important medical procedures. Luckily, this person had connections on the review panel for their coverage and was able to get their surgery covered, but that isn't the case for most people, and no one should have to get such a dangerous surgery solely to access better insurance plans from their employer. This person still had to pay out of pocket for aftercare.

They said:

"If you don't have a complex about still feeling 'fat' for being 'abnormal' for so long, these kinds of processes will SURE give you one! I think it's great that companies are trying to create and promote wellness, but I feel sure there are better ways to go about it than 'threatening' employees in these ways."[75]

It baffles me that our society is still holding on to the false promise of weight loss, despite the fact that the scientific studies that have proven that weight loss doesn't work long-term have been around for the past few decades.

We've abandoned plenty of old paradigms and beliefs over the years; why haven't we abandoned weight loss? Is it because doctors have so much pressure on them to "fix" the o*y problem? Is it because there's still about a 5 percent chance that weight loss could work for some people and medical providers just hope their patients are in that 5 percent? Does the medical industry fear that if the truth of weight loss was revealed, people would give up trying to eat their veggies and exercise regularly? Or is it a lousy excuse to write some patients off?

To me, requirements like the ones discussed above could pose serious issues in terms of body agency, freedom, and privacy. If these types of programs go unchecked, who's to say government-issued meal plans and wellness checks could

---

[75] Anonymous, "Punitive Wellness Programs Are Already Here," *Conscien-Health*, April 4, 2013.

be possible? Could our employers or the government regulate how we eat? If that was the case, what would happen if you failed to follow their regimens? Would you face fines, stricter meal plans, or jail time?

This perhaps pushes the issue too far, but what's to say insurance companies or the government won't go further? The Affordable Care Act made it legal to charge o*e people higher insurance premiums, so to me, that signals the possibility that things could go further if left unchecked.[76]

Diet culture and weight stigma are to blame for all of this. The false belief that anyone who's overweight is unhealthy is why fat people are more likely to face higher insurance premiums and even denial of coverage. The paradigm that thinness equals health has to be smashed. The assumption that someone who is considered overweight is automatically going to be unhealthy and have more costly medical bills is plain wrong.

The European Heart Journal published a twenty-year-long study with United States and European researchers that looked at the metabolic health of 43,265 participants who were considered o*e. The Aerobics Center Longitudinal study discovered that almost 50 percent of the o*e participants were metabolically fit and had no risk of dying earlier than normal weight participants.[77]

---

76   Cedric Jackson, "How Does Health Insurance for Obese People Work?" *Freeway Insurance*, March 13, 2020.

77   Ortega, Francisco B et al. "The intriguing metabolically healthy but obese phenotype: cardiovascular prognosis and role of fitness." *European heart journal* vol. 34,5 (2013): 389-97.

If measuring health was the intention of allowing insurance companies to charge more for "unhealthy" people, why would weight be the main measure of health if weight is not indicative of someone's health? That being said, if insurance companies are charging different prices for people due to assumed higher costs as a result of having "poorer health," where's the line on charging people more due to other health conditions? Could this practice eventually open the door to charging higher premiums for people with other health conditions like addiction, eating disorders, or even genetic conditions?

This kind of legislation, or lack thereof rather, not only causes unfair, arbitrary, excessive costs for people with a higher BMI but also could potentially create a ripple effect in the health care system and lead to higher premiums for other "health" conditions. It's not ethical, and it shouldn't be legal to charge people higher rates because of their weight.

This may sound like a hyperbolic argument, but if weight discrimination is legal and insurance companies have been granted more allowance to charge higher premiums to fat people, what else is going to be allowed in the future?

Weight bias first needs to be addressed in the insurance space. No one should be punished monetarily for living in a bigger body, regardless of their health status.

In addition, employers shouldn't have the autonomy to tell employees what to do with their bodies, regardless of their health concerns. Health is personal and confidential, and it is none of an employer's business. Lastly, weight bias needs to be added to Federal Employment Equal Opportunity laws in order to dismantle weight discrimination in the workplace. Appearance has nothing to do with work performance, and pay should not be affected by your body size. In order to break down fatphobia, we need to start in insurance spaces and the workplace.

CHAPTER 7

FATPHOBIA
AND QUACK DOCTORS

———

A concept our society can sometimes forget is that doctors and health professionals are human too and, by definition, are not infallible. Diet culture is sneaky, and it can fool even the most intelligent, educated people. Doctors are not immune to the virus that is diet culture.

Take Dr. Oz, for example. You may have heard of his show, *The Dr. Oz Show*, or have even seen him on *Oprah* or magazine covers. He has countless published books, millions of weekly viewers, and has made many appearances on the magazines you see while in line at the grocery store that tout results that seem too good to be true. He's promoted raspberry ketones and green coffee bean extract as "miracle" weight loss agents and has even said that a key to living a longer life is having around two hundred orgasms a year.

He's faced a lot of backlash for his extreme convictions in "alternative" medicine, and there's a reason for that. As much as some of us want to have "alternative" options in medicine, alternative medicine is alternative for a reason: It lacks scientific evidence. If homeopathy alternatives were proven to be successful in treating ailments, homeopathy would be considered plain medicine.

Take his coffee bean "miracle cure." At the beginning of one of his shows, Oz asserted, "You may think that magic is make-believe, but this little bean has scientists saying they have found a magic weight-loss cure for every body type. It's green coffee beans, and, when turned into a supplement— this miracle pill can burn fat fast. This is very exciting. And it's breaking news."[78]

If you wanted to know how those coffee beans turned out, the FTC has sued the company for false advertising that promoted the green coffee beans.

The argument for the green coffee bean weight loss cure was that the chlorogenic acid present in green coffee beans aids in limiting glucose absorption. The assumption was not supported by data, so Oz took it upon himself to make his own study, which was conveniently funded by Applied Food Sciences, a company that sold green coffee beans. In his study, people lost a few pounds, but the evidence was debatable. As someone who's in recovery from an eating disorder and had pretty much tried everything to lose weight in her past life, I'd guess that the coffee bean pills work a lot like "fat burners"—you ingest a high amount of caffeine and your

---

[78] Michael Specter, "The Operator: Is the Most Trusted Doctor in America Doing More Harm Than Good?" *New Yorker*, January 28, 2013.

metabolism speeds up a little bit. Your appetite is then suppressed, so you might lose a few pounds but gain them back once you go off them or once your body adjusts to them. You're anxious as heck, probably have trouble sleeping, and sweat profusely from all the caffeine. Taking supplements like that is disordered and, I'd venture to say, not great for you. But television shows love a great breakthrough-quick-fix story, right?

Oz's coffee beans and raspberry ketones didn't last long, though. Congress ripped into him in a hearing in 2014, when a Senate subcommittee questioned many of his claims. Senator Clair McCaskill (D-MO) commented, "I don't get why you need to say this stuff because you know it's not true," after stating dubious claims, such as the raspberry ketone "cure."[79]

At the time, a team of medical researchers investigated the claims Dr. Oz had made on his show and determined that 60 percent of them lacked scientific evidence. Of that, four out of every ten claims Oz made on his show had no scientific basis at all. Not long after that investigation, 1,300 doctors signed a letter calling him "a quack and a fake and a charlatan" whose "advice endangers patients."[80]

Dr. Oz isn't the only one who's fallen off the beaten path of evidence-based medicine, however. Take Ken D. Berry, MD. A quick Google search of him will immediately show his

79   Karen Kaplan, "Real-World Doctors Fact-Check Dr. Oz, and the Results Aren't Pretty," *LA Times*, December 19, 2014.

80   Michael Schein, "Dr. Oz Makes Millions Even Though He's Been Called a 'Charlatan' (and You Should Follow His Lead)," *Forbes*, May 25, 2018.

book about the ketogenic diet and a YouTube video titled "We All Have That 'Skinny' Friend Who Can Eat All the Cake, Bread & Pasta but Never Gains Any Weight. Are They Healthy???"

This guy has over a million YouTube subscribers. Berry has harnessed his own "transformation story" to sell absolutely bogus information to his followers.

His bio on YouYube:

"I used to be a fat, miserable, ignorant doctor, until I slowly discovered the power of removing the slow-poisons of the standard diet, and replacing them with the nourishment of a proper human diet. . . ."[81]

There's a lot to unpack here. First, his fatphobia is glaring. Claiming he was "miserable and ignorant" until he removed "poisons" from his diet? When he says poisons, he means carbohydrates, which, in fact, are our bodies' primary source of energy and are necessary for brain function and a whole lot of other bodily processes. Maybe his information is distorted because his brain is exhausted from trying to run solely on fats.

Second, his remark about being fat could be easily interpreted as a blanket statement that fat people are by default miserable and ignorant and are feeding themselves poison. This language is so harmful and wrong. . . . Carbs are our body's primary source of energy. We need glucose to function. Being fat

---

[81]   Ken D. Berry, YouTube Bio, written on October 8, 2017.

won't be the worst thing to ever happen to us. But according to this doctor, humans just "aren't meant to metabolize carbs."

Somebody get this guy a granola bar.

He demonizes carbs and promotes the ketogenic diet, a diet that was created to reduce seizures in young children with epilepsy that's now been co-opted by diet companies everywhere; the carnivore diet, where you only eat meat; and intermittent fasting, which is a ridiculous excuse to restrict eating and is not necessary at all. For the record, the keto diet isn't meant for adults and is not healthy at all. Our brains and muscles need carbs to function, and if you're having to drink salty bone broth to prevent dehydration on a diet, it's probably not good for you or sustainable (I've been there).

When I did keto before I knew the truth about it, I remember my body giving out on me while teaching a dance cardio class and feeling like I couldn't move my legs because there was so much lactate buildup (that burning sensation you normally feel when working out, but imagine that times 1,000). Lifting weights and doing intense cardio was so difficult on keto; my muscles would almost freeze up and I'd feel so weak that I realized if I couldn't do what I normally can do, this diet was probably not right for me. I would end up binging on carbs at the end of the day because my body needed them—and then I would feel so guilty for "breaking" the diet. Please, don't do keto unless you're a toddler suffering from seizures.

He also touts that fasting is the cheapest way to diet! As if it's healthy to stop eating for extended periods of time. Last time I checked, a lot people go to treatment for that, except it's called an eating disorder.

He has videos named "NEVER Eat Wheat" and asserts that carbs and sugar "weaken" the immune system (more bogusness). I live with privilege in that I don't have any chronic physical health problems, so it's important for me to acknowledge that, but ever since I've been in recovery from an eating disorder, I haven't gotten sick. I eat more carbs and sugar than I ever allowed myself to, I don't deprive myself, and . . . it doesn't look like my immune system is compromised by wheat.

The most concerning part about his social media presence is that people follow him and take his words for fact, since after all, he is a doctor. He retweeted a post commenting "Ive never read something more true than this" that said:

"200 years ago, before refrigerators, microwaves & Uber Eats; 'time-restricted feeding' was 'eating,' 'Whole food plant based' was 'summer/autumn,' 'Keto/carnivore' was 'winter/spring,' 'Alternate day fasting' was 'it got away,' Yet, dietitians call them eating disorders."[82]

Yeah, dietitians call them eating disorders because they are the ones who are educated in nutrition. They know what they're talking about and are way more qualified than you are

---

[82] Tro. Kalayjian, "200 years ago, before refrigerators, microwaves & Uber Eats; 'time-restricted feeding' was 'eating,' 'Whole food plant based' was 'summer/autumn,' 'Keto/carnivore' was 'winter/spring,' 'Alternate day fasting' was 'it got away,' Yet, dietitians call them eating disorders." Twitter, March 12, 2020.

in the nutrition department. There's a reason people didn't live very long two hundred years ago.

This sounds like a rant, and in a lot of ways, it is, but I think that in order to talk about fatphobia and medical care and where they intersect, it's really important to look at more extreme examples of doctors out there who are campaigning against the "fight against o*y" in ways that are completely harmful, false, and would result in the diagnosis of an eating disorder in a thin person. With an MD comes responsibility, and unfortunately, not everyone on Earth is responsible, and no one is perfect.

It's also important to note that many people promote whatever diet worked for them and assume that if they succeeded with it, others will too. For all we know, this man struggled with his weight and felt his own shame around being bigger and now projects that into other people, because that was his experience. He could very likely have an unhealthy relationship with food.

We can't talk about fatphobia without calling out fearmongering, diet culture-infested bogusness that is inherently fatphobic and meant to sell you something. Diet culture profits off insecurities and fears and preys on the vulnerable. You might see it on your morning news specials, in ads on your phone, or in your doctor's office, often presented as "weight management."

In today's world, if you have any sort of certification next to your name, a lot of people believe what you say. When I was in college, I was a certified fitness instructor, taught at several gyms, and ran a personal training and meal coaching business that I had no business running. I had some whack one-day certificate on eating "whole foods plant based," and called that a nutrition certification. The people who trained me claimed they reversed cancer in themselves by eating this way—once again, crazy and terrible misinformation. I lasted about two weeks eating like that until I realized my body just isn't meant to not have meat. Some people choose to go without meat for moral or environmental reasons, and that's great, as long as you're not compromising your relationship with food or feeling deprived in any way.

I point out my own past mistakes to say that a lot of us have been there. I take accountability for my past preaching about unsustainable dieting and fitness plans. When I was sick with my eating disorder, I really thought I was helping people gain confidence and reach their weight loss goals, but I probably caused more harm long-term teaching disordered eating habits to others.

I understand where these people are coming from because I've done it myself. Aside from making money off of it, doctors who tout ridiculous diets and weight loss products often genuinely believe they are helping people.

I say this to highlight that people aren't usually trying to be malicious when making ridiculous claims. I'm not here to point fingers or blame people for whatever it is they're doing. Almost all of us have some level of internalized fatphobia solely from growing up in this culture and subconsciously holding on to the messaging we've gotten from existing in our society. That's okay.

Now that we can name it, it's time to take matters into our own hands and unlearn the fatphobic beliefs that have been shoved down our throats all our life. It's time to take our power back. I hope that one day people of all sizes can live in peace and non-judgment from others, and from themselves. Like I've said before, it's not our fault we grew up in this society, but it is our responsibility to challenge our beliefs and stand up against ridiculous, fatphobic practices, whether it be bogus information from doctors like Oz and Berry, comments on our sister's weight by Aunt Betty, or downright discrimination in the workplace, in medicine, or in social settings. Together, we can work to debunk public figures' misinformation and call out diet culture for what it is—fatphobic, unethical, and lacking in scientific evidence.[83]

---

[83] Jon C. Tilburt, Megan Allyse, and Frederic W. Hafferty, "The Case of Dr. Oz: Ethics, Evidence, and Does Professional Self-Regulation Work?" *AMA J Ethics*, 19 no. 2, (2017):199–206.

CHAPTER 8

CHILDREN
AND FATPHOBIA

———

Should doctors put kids on diets? Do we need to discuss weight with children? If our kid comes to us upset about their body, what should we do? How can we make doctors' offices a safer, fatphobia-free space for kids, and how can we do that in our homes?

We'll tackle these difficult questions in this chapter by hearing a friend, Candice, share her experience with doctors as a kid, and later we'll explore Dana Suchow's take on navigating body image, weight, and fatphobia with kids. Dana is an award-winning speaker and educator on children's body image.

The following story is in Candice' words.

"I was about five years old when the doctor started getting on me about the foods I ate.

"I was awkward. I had kinky, frizzy, yet brushed out hair and straight-across bangs (my parents didn't know how to handle my hair) and was as uncomfortable in my skin as a budding middle schooler going through puberty before anyone else.

"Boys picked on me, nagging about my 'puffy hair.' They took my crayons. Some kids called me fat, and I believed them.

"So at a ripe age of five, I already felt pretty down on myself. I felt different from other kids. I had plenty of friends, but I didn't look like your typical skinny-straight-blonde-hair schoolgirl at my school, and I hated that.

"One Friday, my mom picked my sister and me up to take us to our annual physical after school.

After the initial weight, height, and vital tests, Dr. Jason asked, 'So, what does your eating look like?'

"My mom responded 'Candice is a picky eater. She eats Eggo waffles for breakfast, peanut butter and jellies for lunch every day, and will only eat chicken fingers at restaurants. She does eat fruit. Her sister Camila will eat anything, though!'

"I squirm on the table in silence, waiting in nervousness in my plaid jumper that's already a little too tight. I have a chocolate stain on my white blouse sleeve, because every Tuesday I would get chicken nuggets and ice cream for lunch, and apparently preferred to use my shirt to wipe my face.

"I was picky because I had already picked up on the idea of what's 'healthy' and what's not at home and chose to not eat pasta, burgers, buns, etc. because I thought they were 'bad.' I already had guilt about the food I liked, so I thought if I avoided the other 'bad' foods, I wouldn't be *as* bad. At age five, I was afraid of food. At dinner, I'd hear 'See Candice, Camila will eat the ___, why can't you?'

"It made me feel like I wasn't good enough, but I didn't know any better and saw my parents' dieting and weighing themselves as a regular thing people do. My parents didn't know any better either; they wanted the best for me, and at the time, they worried for my health.

"'Well she's going to need to branch out and start eating healthier foods. . . . She could be at risk for developing diabetes,' Dr. Jason scolded. 'I have some ideas for you on helping her branch out, Mrs. Thompson.'

"Next thing I knew, a week later my mom had drawn up a chart with fruits and vegetables with points assigned to eating each one and presented it to me when I got home from school one day.

"'Dr. Jason came up with this idea, if you try anything on this list, I'll give you points, and accumulated points will count towards new toys you'd like!'

"Now I know what you might be thinking—either, 'This is crazy,' or, 'What a great idea to get my kids to eat healthier!' Either way, don't do it.

"My mom did what she thought was best for me. A doctor told her that her daughter was at risk for developing diabetes and gave her this idea to get me to eat different foods. She was doing her best, and it is *not* her fault that it may have subtly begun to distort my relationship with food. What mother wouldn't listen to a highly respected pediatrician?"

"I don't blame my mother one bit for that entire situation," Candice says. "She loved me, and worried I'd get sick if I didn't change my habits. She's not responsible for coming up with an incentivized idea like that, my doctor was."

What Dr. Jason didn't tell her, and probably didn't know, was that a child is 242 times more likely to develop an eating disorder than he or she is to develop diabetes.[84]

But that's not what we hear in the news, or in the doctor's office.

We hear that type 2 diabetes is a rampant problem. I've personally seen so many fearmongering billboards on road trips that claim that "83 Million People are Pre-Diabetic. Guy Stuck-in-Traffic." Where did that number even come from, and what percentage of those people actually develop type 2 diabetes? Although pre-diabetes is a real diagnosis, a lot of the numbers used in these campaigns are claims that people are undiagnosed, which can totally be true. However, intimidating people with these stats doesn't help anything.

---

[84] L. Bacon and L. Aphramor, *Body Respect: What Conventional Health Books Get Wrong, Leave Out, and Just Plain Fail to Understand about Weight.* (Dallas: BenBella Books, 2014).

We don't hear that someone dies from an eating disorder every fifty-two minutes.[85]

(When I started writing this book, the death rate was every sixty-two minutes. That terrifies me.)

We definitely don't hear that the number of people with eating disorders in bigger or straight-sized bodies doubles that of people who are underweight.

No, we hear that we'll get diabetes if we eat too much sugar. We're told that o*y is a nationwide crisis that we must solve before everyone dies of cardiovascular problems, diabetes, and hypertension.

We're all afraid to be fat because we know how fat people are seen and treated. We live in a society that sees fat people as inferior, lazy, out of control and believe fat people are personally responsible for being fat. We are obsessed with thinness, we only see thin bodies in the media, and expect our bodies to obey our dieting, despite the fact that in reality, people aren't as thin as the media portrays. The average size of a woman in America is a 14, yet the media we consume doesn't portray that.[86]

Dr. Jason isn't a registered dietician, and neither are primary care doctors, unless you happen to see someone with both credentials. Doctors take maybe three nutrition classes through-

---

[85] Striped, "Report: Economic Costs of Eating Disorders. Harvard T.H. Chan School of Public Health," (June 2020).

[86] Pamela Peeke, "Just What IS an Average Woman's Size Anymore?" *WebMD*, January 25, 2010.

out the entire course of medical school. They're seen as the experts in eating, but they're really not. They went to school to diagnose health issues, diseases, and prescribe medicine to treat them. They've been pressured to take on the task of advising people on their diet when they weren't trained to do so.

Doctors are taught that what they prescribe for someone with anorexia is also what they prescribe for people who are obese, despite the fact that 95–97 percent of diets fail because genetics, social determinants, and many other factors play too large a role for us to be able to successfully control our body size long-term.[87] It's not their fault they weren't given ample education on the topic, but . . . that's what registered dietitians are for.

So while Candice's mom and her doctor were doing what they thought was the right thing to do, Candice started fearing foods and seeing foods as morally "good" or "bad."

Candice states, "This was the beginning of a voice in my head that slowly grew louder and louder, and eventually developed into an eating disorder when I experienced more stressful and traumatic events in my adolescence."

Adults aren't the only people who struggle with body image and food; kids do, too. When parents or doctors project fears of being fat on children, they absorb that information and take it as fact; they don't understand diet culture like adults can.

---

[87]   A. Stunkard and M. McLaren-Hume, "The Results of Treatment for Obesity: A Review of the Literature and Report of a Series," *AMA Arch Intern Med.*, 103, no. 1, (1959):79–85.

Dana Suchow, child body image expert and award-winning speaker and educator, weighed in on the topic of weight talk at the doctor and shared how providers and parents can raise body-confident children by ditching the weight talk and empowering children to listen to their bodies. Dana speaks at schools and works with kids, but the majority of the work she does is with parents, teachers, and caregivers.

During our interview, Dana shared some insight that really resonated with me:

"I'll go to a workshop and we start talking, and after half an hour during the workshop, what really comes out is people's own internal trauma, their own internal biases, their own internal fatphobia, racism, sexism, whatever it is that they have. And then they start seeing how,

'Well okay so this is how I talk about bodies. And now I can see my child picking up the same thing,' or you know when a child comes to a parent and says, 'I feel fat, I don't like my body,' what happens is the parent immediately responds in a panic and goes, 'Oh my gosh, my child is going to live through the same exact traumas and bullying that I did.

"And so, I believe truly that almost all parents and caregivers are coming from a place of love and protection."

This idea that adults project their own fears and traumas onto children isn't new; it's a totally normal phenomenon, especially within the framework of parenting. This "protective projection" isn't solely reserved for parents, however.

Combine internalized fatphobia from society with years of medical school education and anti-o*y campaigns, and you have an army of very fearful health care providers who have been tasked with having to offer advice to children who are considered overweight. Sounds like a pretty difficult endeavor, doesn't it?

Of course, this isn't to say that every single healthcare provider holds fatphobic sentiments, but it's imprudent to make the assumption that every provider has had education around weight bias. Our current medical system's framework is inherently fatphobic, as we've seen in previous chapters.

Suchow suggests that as a caregiver or provider, before you speak to a child about their body, pause and imagine yourself in their shoes. How would you have wanted to be spoken to as a child? If you were young, how would you have felt if you doctor, mother, or relative told you your body wasn't okay the way it was? Maybe that's happened to you. How did that event make you feel? Did it help improve your health? I'm going to bet that it didn't.

The reality is, kids aren't supposed to be on diets, they and shouldn't be restricting their calories at all. They're growing! Putting kids on diets can stunt development and growth; I've seen it through friends who wrestled in grade school and had to heavily restrict to "make weight" for meets. They blame their wrestling days for their lack of growth in middle and high school. Adolescent kids eat a lot for a reason; they're hungry and they're growing.

If you are a provider, before you talk about a child's weight (if you *really* have to), tell the child you need to speak with the parent about some billing information (for example), and speak to the parent in private where the child can't hear. Suchow emphasizes that no child should be a part of a weight conversation, much less be in the same room as one. Children's brains aren't fully developed, and therefore, they cannot process these kinds of conversations in the context they're meant to be in (consider this: you may take the comment "you would benefit from losing x pounds" as it is, while a child may take that comment as "you're unlovable and not good enough because you need to lose x pounds").

Dana explained that it's important to recognize that children's bodies change drastically as they're growing. She used her brother as an example.

"My brother was five years younger than me, so I remember my brother when he was going through puberty, he was like an accordion. He would shoot up like a beanstalk, and then he would be chubby, and then he'd shoot up again and that was just how he grew."

Kids' bodies are going to change a lot as they develop. Normalize the idea that their bodies are growing and will change and look different, and often, these changes are a part of getting strong and growing up. Assure the child that it's normal and healthy for their bodies to change.

Before you bring up weight around a child, Dana advises adults to remember that "No matter what their size, weight, whatever it is . . . shame and anxiety and embarrassment will never work to promote change in a child [or] in any of us."

Did bullying, weight comments, or the like ever help anyone? Were you ever talked to about your weight in a negative way, and did it go well and strengthen your trust and love for someone else?

Shame doesn't help anyone, and it especially doesn't help kids.

I had an experience at a yoga workshop years ago that I think is a helpful story to turn to when thinking about approaching children with topics like body image and body size. If you're a doctor, a parent, or a caregiver of some sort, consider the following inner child exercise before talking to a child about their weight.

* * *

When I taught group exercise, I remember one weekend a group of us attended a fitness conference in Asheville, NC, that offered continuing education credits. We took two vans, and the van I took didn't have any supervisors in it, only fitness instructors. Someone had brought a bunch of cookies, which led to a guilt-filled conversation that turned into one I wasn't expecting.

My coworker Chanel had reluctantly eaten two cookies and wouldn't stop talking about the guilt of eating "straight sugar." I had eaten seven.

She started opening up: "When I was in middle school, my parents sent me away to fat camp."

Everyone was in shock. "You went to fat camp?"

"Yeah, I actually went to fat camp. I lost eighty pounds by cycling. It was horrible, but that's kind of why I love teaching Spin so much; I lost so much weight from it. I definitely have a lot of anxiety around food, and I know I kind of obsess over eating healthy, but I just don't ever want to go through what I went through as a kid again. I hated myself, and I was bullied so much."

Another instructor, Emily, chimed in. She'd been bullied as a kid for her size and was in the depths of bulimia, but couldn't figure out how to get out of the vicious restrict, binge, and purge cycle.

Then another instructor chimed in and revealed their own struggles with disordered eating.

Then another one shared, "I was always bigger, and when I came to school here, where so many people are thin, I decided if I dedicated all my time to teaching exercise classes, my body type would be more acceptable.

"I remember teaching three classes a day sometimes; I lived at the gym. I had no life. I was alone and miserable, and I stopped getting my period for a while. I got help and am doing so much better now, but I still struggle with orthorexia. It's just so hard to be in the fitness scene and not let the culture faze you, you know?"

The van got really quiet. That was the same month I had begun to realize my own issues with food and exercise, but I was still too ashamed to say anything about it. I had binged all weekend.

One of the workshops at the conference was a yoga meditation and education session called "The Issues Are in Our Tissues." The woman who led the group had been sober for several years and discussed how trauma gets stored in the body; our bodies remember it, tighten up, and carry traumatic experiences in our hips, back, neck, and it usually presents itself as tightness or pain.

At the end of the session, we all closed our eyes, got comfortable, and took part in a guided meditation by the leader. I don't recall every detail of the meditation, so consider this a paraphrased, shortened version of it:

"Close your eyes and imagine a beautiful meadow. You're walking through it, sun beaming down on your face, breeze flowing through your hair, and you notice a stream. The grass is lush and green surrounding it, and the dandelions are in full bloom. Hear the quiet rush of water as it runs down the nook. You take a deep breath and inhale the fresh air.

"You begin to approach a small child. That child is you, at age three. Take [his/her/their] hand. Kneel down next to her so you're at eye level.

"Tell her how wonderful she is. Tell her that everything turned out fine for her. Tell her that she is enough, just the way she is. You don't have to be perfect to be loved, dear. You're doing great, and you're going to be an amazing person one day; you already are.

"Give your child self a hug and tell her you'll always be there for her. It's time to go now.

When you're ready, give yourself a hug, and slowly open your eyes. That child is within you, and it's your job to protect her and tell her she's more than good enough, just the way she is."

Although it's not nearly as powerful over text, we all ended the meditation in tears. I was sobbing. I felt so much pain for my younger self, who thought that because she was different, she wasn't good enough.

If you're a provider and happen to have a young patient whose BMI falls into a higher-than-normal category, before bringing it up in front of the child, picture your younger, child self being told their weight is higher than what's healthy. Step into their shoes. Is it helpful or harmful? Chances are, it's the latter.

Something important to remember when interacting with children is that they're completely dependent on adults; they need caregivers for their survival. Dana Suchow reminded me in our conversation that children are going to do whatever they can to keep an adult's protection and love. Children look up to adults; they have authority. Doctors have authority, too. When kids are approached with weight talks, diet talks, and the idea that their body needs to be changed, Dana added that "We're setting them up for a lifetime of needing approval, for a lifetime of fear of being the 'other,' and feeling like they have to completely change their bodies to be accepted."

Do you want that for your child or patient?

If you're a parent or provider who's worried about your child's health, before you jump to conclusions out of fear, check the reality of the situation. In 2014–2015, there were five thousand eight hundred children with type 2 diabetes in the US.[88]

According to Census.gov, in 2014, there were approximately 82,108,087 children under the age of nineteen in the United States.[89]

So even though the CDC warns us that 1 in 3 children are at risk for developing type 2 because 1 in 3 children are considered overweight, that warning doesn't really add up when you look at the numbers.

While we're talking about it, childhood diabetes is a commonly feared illness that is often all over the news media. We see this stuff in nationwide campaigns against childhood o*y, like former first lady Michelle Obama's campaign, *Let's Move*. We have a White House Task Force on Childhood O*y. Yet, over sixteen million children struggle with hunger each year in the United States, and as a result, about 1 in 5 children go hungry each year.[90] In my opinion, for being as wealthy of a country as the US, that's a much more worrisome statistic than stats on o*y.

---

[88] "Statistics About Diabetes," American Diabetes Association, Accessed April 17, 2020.

[89] "Mid-year Population by Youth Age Groups and Sex - Custom Region - United States," United States Census: International Programs, Accessed April 17, 2020.

[90] "Facts About Child Hunger in America," *No Kid Hungry*, Accessed April 18, 2020.

We need to educate children on how to separate the fatphobic, diet culture-ridden messaging in our society from reality as they develop. This might look like this:

A commercial comes on about a diet program, or it makes a joke about weight.

Caregiver to child: "Sam, those ads aren't accurate. Bodies need lots of different types of food to be strong and healthy. Our body size doesn't determine how healthy we are! That company just wants to make money by profiting off of people's insecurities. That is diet culture, and we don't listen to that silly stuff here. All bodies are good bodies, and I'll love you no matter what you look like or what size you wear."

I remember the next generation food pyramid was developed during the time of the campaign. The food pyramid became "MyPlate," the new USDA standard for dietary guidelines. I remember using the app in middle school to track my calories (sounds healthy right?).

Looking back, I'm surprised there weren't notifications that would tell you if you ate too little or needed to eat more of a certain food group. I also don't recall any age controls for using the app. Food for thought, USDA.

With social media, access to the internet, and what's taught in schools so early on today, we have to help our kids filter out the truth from the bogusness. If you ever come across a fatphobic ad around your child, call it out and help them understand that body discrimination is wrong, and so is the media's misrepresentation of body diversity.

When health care providers and parents are bombarded with fearmongering messages about childhood o*y and childhood diabetes, it's easy to feed into that fear and project it onto children. This won't help them, no matter how big or small they might be.

Body size "health concerns" may be well-intended, but they often result in shame. Dr. Brene Brown defines shame as "the intensely painful feeling or experience of believing that we are flawed and therefore unworthy of love and belonging."[91] Whether we mean to or not, commenting negatively on children's body size or food choices can cause shame. Often times, these comments come from the internalized shame around our own bodies. Maybe we were shamed for our food choices and taught we must eat or look a certain way to be accepted, and passing it on to those around us was our way of helping others cope with society as we did. But did all that shame really help?

Rather than shaming children for their food choices or body size, we must empower them to look inward in terms of how they understand health. We have to teach them that health has nothing to do with appearance.

Suchow suggests that when speaking about exercise, talk about building strong muscles and bones so they can carry their backpack with heavy books when they're older. Talk about how mental health is important, and how expressing their feelings is a healthy and normal part of life. Allow

---

[91]   Kathy Slattengren, "Publicly or Privately Shaming Harms Kids," *Priceless Parenting*, Accessed April 18, 2020.

all foods, and rather than labeling foods as healthy and unhealthy, talk about how variety is good for our health.

Jennifer Anderson, MSPH, RDN, also known as @kids.eat. in.color on Instagram, has great graphics for these types of conversations. In one post, a graphic reads, "May not help: Apples are good for you," versus, "May help a lot: Red food gives you a strong heart," and lists several examples.

In order to break the cycle of fatphobia in our society, we must empower our children to reject the idea that one type of body is superior to another. We must teach them that health is a holistic, complex thing that has nothing to do with what size we wear or what we look like. Help your children see the truth behind diet culture messaging in media and give them the tools to listen to their bodies. How freeing would it be if their generation rejects the narrative that thin is king? Give your patient or child permission to live free from the shackles of the weight-normative narrative.

CHAPTER 9

THE DANGERS OF GASTRIC BYPASS SURGERY

This chapter is in no way meant to shame anyone who's had weight loss surgery or plans to; I'm a firm believer in your body, your choice. It's more than understandable to want to be smaller in a world that treats us accordingly based on our appearance. For some people, it's a life-changing surgery that does improve their well-being.

However, as much as weight loss surgeries are advertised as safe and effective, there are some complications that go along with it that aren't talked about enough. A lot of current literature on weight loss surgery emphasizes its benefits and tends to minimize the risks (hi, diet culture). My hope is to shed light on some of the possible dangers involved in such a drastic surgery and to explore why our society continues to uphold surgery as the best option possible for people in bigger bodies.

Katie Logue, twenty-six at the time, decided to undergo gastric bypass surgery in 2010. She was at her wits' end with weight loss. She'd tried every diet she could with no avail, was considered "on the fast track" to diabetes and heart disease according to her doctors, and wanted to grow her family, but believed she couldn't get pregnant at her weight. Katie wanted to be more present for her son and made the decision to have weight loss surgery, as it seemed like the only choice she had left to get her life back.

Within six months following surgery, Katie lost 100 pounds. But as the weight continued to fall off, Katie began to experience some stomach pain and nausea. When she contacted her surgeon about her symptoms, Katie was written off.

"Looking as good as you do, you must be pregnant."

Her surgeon gave her a pregnancy test and left.

Unfortunately, her surgeon was wrong, and not long after the visit, Katie was rushed into emergency surgery for intussusception (the inversion of one portion of the intestine within another), a small bowel obstruction, and a perforated ulcer.

This was the beginning of a long battle with gastrointestinal issues, emergency surgeries, and chronic pain for Katie.

Months after Katie's surgery, she was rushed again to the trauma center at a local hospital. She was having the same problem she had months prior and had to undergo another surgery:

"Once again I was diagnosed with the rare condition known as intussusception, and once again I found myself in surgery to correct the intussusception. I have now had three small bowel resections."

A week later, Katie had a pill lodged in her stomach that had to be surgically removed, but her surgeon never told her that was that case. Katie only learned that the pill was the culprit years later because she requested her medical records and found a packet that described what had really happened that time.

Katie was sent home that night with a visiting nurse and a feeding tube, hair falling out, malnourished, ten months post-operation, at age twenty-seven.

"My condition was grave. At five foot seven I weighed a mere 112 pounds; so sick and malnourished, my hair was falling out despite the feeding tube, which had become lodged in my abdomen and would ultimately require yet another surgery to be removed."

Then she had her appendix removed.

Next thing she knew, Katie was uncontrollably vomiting and couldn't leave her bed for days. When the vomiting didn't stop, she was rushed to the hospital and had open surgery and later learned she had an ulcer that perforated in two places and had leaked toxic fluids into her system. Boston's Chief of Surgery told her she was lucky to be alive.

Katie had a respite from health issues for a short few years. Aside from chronic nausea and pain, there were no surgeries or hospital visits.

However, she said, "Since July I have spent more time in the hospital than out."

Katie's been diagnosed with an ovarian cyst, irritable bowel syndrome, gastritis, and "nearly every GI condition possible."

By age thirty-two, she was considered infertile by doctors. One of the reasons she had the surgery was to be able to have more children. But now, she can't—plus, her hair is falling out, she has an ulcer, and lives with chronic pain and nausea.

Katie thought she'd "get her life back" through surgery, but instead, she's out of work, her eight-year-old son helps her carry things because he recognizes she's ill and in pain, she can't have kids anymore, and deals with chronic nausea and pain.

In an article she wrote about her story with surgery, she said:

"Gastric bypass robbed me of more than my fertility. I now live in continual fear that something will go wrong and I will once again be at the mercy of whatever surgeon has my case thrown at him. Bob Seger says it best in his hit song 'Against the Wind' when he says, 'I wish I didn't know now what I didn't know then.' Oh how I wish . . ."[92]

---

[92] Katie Logue, "When Gastric Bypass Surgery Goes Horribly Wrong," *Her View from Home*, Accessed May 8, 2020.

Gastric bypass and bariatric surgery seem to be the gold standard in the medical field as the most effective way to treat o*y for years, but is it really that safe?

Weight loss surgery has gained popularity in the last few decades. In the early 1990s, only sixteen thousand people underwent surgery.[93] Fast forward to 2017, two hundred twenty-eight thousand people underwent surgery, and that number is slowly climbing.[94]

Although the death rate has declined in recent years, health risks are still involved.

According to the Mayo Clinic, risks include:

- infection,
- excessive bleeding,
- blood clots,
- lung problems,
- leaks in the gastrointestinal system,
- and death.

Long term risks include:

- bowel obstruction,

93 "Information on Bariatric Surgery," *US News & World Report*, Last Reviewed January 8, 2010.

94 Amber Hamilton, "New Study Finds Most Bariatric Surgeries Performed in Northeast, and Fewest in South Where Obesity Rates are Highest, and Economies are Weakest," *American Society for Metabolic and Bariatric Surgery*, November 15, 2018.

- dumping syndrome (diarrhea, flushing, lightheadedness, nausea, vomiting),
- gallstones,
- hernias,
- hypoglycemia,
- malnutrition,
- ulcers,
- vomiting,
- acid reflux,
- the need for a second procedure,
- and death.

Mayo Clinic warned that weight-loss surgeries "don't always work as well as you might have hoped." It warns that "if a weight loss procedure doesn't work well or stops working, you may not lose weight and you may develop serious health problems."[95]

Recently, indirect consequences of gastric bypass surgery have become more prevalent. For example, drug- and alcohol-related deaths tripled in patients who underwent gastric bypass surgery, or Roux-en-Y, which is the most popular weight loss surgery. In the operation, 95 percent of the stomach is removed. This takes away most of the alcohol receptors in the stomach, leaving the liver to do all the heavy lifting when metabolizing alcohol (usually, alcohol is metabolized in the stomach, then in the liver). In a study comparing adults who've had the surgery compared to adults who haven't, on average, 89 out of 100,000 patients who had the surgery died of drug overdoses or alcoholic diseases, while

---

[95] "Bariatric Surgery," *Mayo Clinic*, January 22, 2020.

30.5 out of 100,000 of the general population died of the same causes.[96]

Although studies say that the risk of death has drastically reduced in recent years (in 2005, 1 in 50 people died from surgery), the risks are still present.[97] Just last year, a woman died of malnutrition in the years following her surgery. Kimberly Wall, mother of three, reported that she regretted the surgery once she noticed she became more anxious and depressed over time and had so much trouble eating that she was unable to walk at one point. She passed after being hospitalized for a week due to heart failure as a result of malnutrition.[98]

A simple Google search of "Weight Loss Surgery Complications Forum" will take you to an Obesity Help forum that has volumes of complaints of complications reported from people who've had the surgery, ranging from sphincter closing, feeling pressure and "stuck food," pain, suture erosion, vomiting, chronic nausea, bowel obstruction, ulcers, blind loop syndrome, and more.

Yet, when searching for the risks associated with the surgery, some of the top articles that come up claim that the surgery decreases risks of death and has very few side effects. Many people who've gotten the surgery do not hold the same sentiment.

[96] Donna Siegfried, "Rates of Drug-, Alcohol-Linked Death Triple after Weight Loss Surgery," *US News*, June 20, 2019.

[97] Tatiana Morales, "Gastric Bypass Surgery Gone Bad," *CBS News*, January 21, 2005.

[98] Gabby Landsverk, "A Woman Died of Malnutrition after Weight-Loss Surgery Led Her Lose 250 Pounds over 10 Years," *Insider*, October 18, 2019.

In a world where thinness is the sole sign of health, it's only fair to explore the downsides of a surgery whose risks often aren't discussed enough. This isn't to say that everyone who gets the surgery has all of these issues, but it's important to talk to your doctor and make sure you aren't at risk, and that the surgeon is experienced and has had successful outcomes in past patients if it's something you're considering.

It's not right that people aren't equipped with the stats of side effects, risks, and possible complications that can lead to death when preparing for such an invasive surgery. Like I said, however, if it's something you've looked into, I respect your decision. It's an incredibly difficult and complex topic. My main concern is the ethics behind doctors and surgeons possibly omitting some of the complications and risks when discussing the surgery with patients. My hope is that in the future, cutting out parts of organs isn't a second-in-line (first being diet and exercise) "treatment" for being fat. We shouldn't have to feel like we need to massively change our internal systems surgically to be "healthier," but we can thank general fatphobia for that.

PART 3:

ADVOCATING FOR YOURSELF, DISROBING YOUR OWN FATPHOBIA, AND PRACTICING WEIGHT-INCLUSIVE MEDICINE

CHAPTER 10

HAES AND WHY
IT WORKS

We now know that using weight loss as the primary approach to improving health hasn't been effective or sustainable, so what should be done instead?

In this chapter, we'll look at the Health at Every Size method of treatment and compare it to the weight loss method. Jonah, whose name was changed for his privacy, dealt with knee issues for a while and received various types of treatment. Let's look at two different examples from his experience and examine the efficacy of each.

EXAMPLE 1:

Jonah has recently taken up running each morning before work and lives in a bigger body. He began to suffer from knee pain and asked his doctor about it at his annual checkup.

Jonah's doctor advised him to lose weight and noted, "Since you're heavier, you're naturally going to have added pressure to your joints. Lose fifty pounds and get back to me on how that knee pain is."

Jonah went home and researched some ways to lose weight. He began a restrictive diet that cut out a lot of food groups and started tracking his calories. He kept running despite his knee pain. He stopped going out to his weekly dinners with friends to avoid certain foods. Jonah rapidly lost weight and started experiencing insomnia, which he didn't really understand. He lost all sex drive and noticed his hair was thinning slightly. He hit a weight loss plateau, and his hunger started to skyrocket. He'd find himself binging in the middle of the night, sleep-deprived and starving, and would shame himself into "starting over" the next day. He realized if he went over the restrictive calorie limit he began his diet on, he'd gain weight back. However, he couldn't live off of that small of a number of calories anymore. Jonah's weight came back, plus more, and his knee pain became so excruciating that he gave up exercising, defeated and ashamed of failing the weight loss game.

EXAMPLE 2:

Jonah suffered from knee pain and asked his doctor what he could do to relieve it. Jonah's doctor referred him to a physical therapist. With the PT, he went through exercises that were tailored to his body's abilities, focused on strengthening muscle imbalances and weaknesses, and after working through his set of exercises for a few months, his knee pain was almost gone. He continues to incorporate some of his physical therapy exercises into his warm-up before he works out and makes sure he gives his body the rest it needs.

His physical therapist told him, "Because of the way your bones are structured, running is going to strain your knees. Instead of running, try walking, swimming, or using the elliptical instead of the treadmill to reduce stress on your joints. Make sure to give your body time to recover between workouts, as too much high-intensity movement too often can trigger your knee pain. Moderation is key."

The stark difference between the examples are evident. Losing weight wasn't going to solve Jonah's current issue of dealing with knee pain long-term. Sure, he went on a diet and initially lost some weight, but the weight eventually came back, and his knees were so damaged he quit exercising all together.

In addition, the method in the first example didn't examine Jonah's exercise behaviors or the strength imbalances that may have caused the pain in the first place. In the second example, Jonah's behaviors, body structure, and weaknesses were taken into consideration. Jonah now knows that running by nature is too hard on his joints for his specific build, so he swims, walks, or uses the elliptical instead now. He's addressed his muscle imbalances through physical therapy and can now continue his exercise habits with sustainability and joint health in mind. In the second example, Jonah's doctor supported his health by getting him the help he really needed, and now Jonah can move his body without pain.

Example 1 is the weight normative approach: a popular way our society focuses on weight loss as an end-all, be-all cure to ailments. Example 2 is a rudimentary example of Health at Every Size.

Maybe you've heard of Health at Every Size, maybe you haven't. Lindo Bacon, PhD, author of *Health At Every Size: The Surprising Truth About Your Weight, Body Respect: What Conventional Health Books Get Wrong, Leave Out, and Just Plain Fail to Understand about Weight* and *Radical Belonging: How to Survive and Thrive in an Unjust World (While Transforming it for the Better)*, has pioneered dismantling the weight normative approach and encourages people to treat their bodies with the love and respect it deserves, sans dieting and self-harming behaviors. The weight normative approach is the antiquated belief that losing weight is sustainable and works to improve health, regardless of other factors, including but not limited to the physical and mental ramifications of long-term restriction. It's the approach that our health system still uses, even though countless studies done over the past few decades have proven that dieting doesn't work.

What exactly is HAES? The following excerpt from Dr. Bacon's work illustrates the main ideas behind Health at Every Size:

> *Let's face facts. We've lost the war on obesity. Fighting fat hasn't made the fat go away. And being thinner, even if we knew how to successfully accomplish it, will not necessarily make us healthier or happier. The war on obesity has taken its toll.*

> *Extensive "collateral damage" has resulted: Food and body preoccupation, self-hatred, eating disorders, discrimination, poor health, etc. Few of us are at peace with our bodies, whether because we're fat or because we fear becoming fat.*

Health at Every Size is the new peace movement.

It supports people of all sizes in addressing health directly by adopting healthy behaviors. It is an inclusive movement, recognizing that social characteristics, such as our size, race, national origin, sexuality, gender, disability status, and other attributes are assets and acknowledges and challenges the structural and systemic forces that impinge on living well.[99]

HAES has five principles:

1. **Weight Inclusivity:** Accept and respect the inherent diversity of body shapes and sizes and reject the idealizing or pathologizing of specific weights.
2. **Health Enhancement:** Support health policies that improve and equalize access to information and services and personal practices that improve human well-being, including attention to individual physical, economic, social, spiritual, emotional, and other needs.
3. **Respectful Care**: Acknowledge our biases and work to end weight discrimination, weight stigma, and weight bias. Provide information and services from an understanding that socioeconomic status, race, gender, sexual orientation, age, and other identities impact weight stigma and support environments that address these inequities.
4. **Eating for Well-being:** Promote flexible, individualized eating based on hunger, satiety, nutritional needs, and

---

[99] "HAES Includes the Following Basic Components," HAES Community, last reviewed 2020.

pleasure rather than any externally regulated eating plan focused on weight control.

5. **Life-Enhancing Movement:** Support physical activities that allow people of all sizes, abilities, and interests to engage in enjoyable movement to the degree that they choose.[100]

Although a lot of it may sound obvious, instituting HAES principles into your life can be the most freeing and transformative form of self-care as it promotes healthful behaviors without the baggage of diet culture and cultural messaging we've been fed all our lives. HAES recognizes all the nuances and factors that play into overall health and takes into consideration oppressive systems in our society that also impact one's health.

HAES founder Dr. Bacon has spent decades studying and researching HAES, and the results of his studies demonstrate this:

Pressuring someone into losing weight only worsens health long-term. Encouraging people to eat nutritious foods, move their bodies in a way that works for them, treat their body with love and respect, listen to its needs, rest, and focus on building connections that support emotional well-being sees far more rewarding results than the weight-normative approach.

The largest contributor to health is not weight; it's what we call social determinants of health. Social determinants

---

[100] "HAES® Principles," ASDAH: Association for Size Diversity and Health, last reviewed 2020.

include socioeconomic status, education, physical environments, social and support networks, access to health care, and family life, as well as race, gender orientations, and any identity that can cause stigma or discrimination. Dr. Bacon shared that these factors eclipse eating and exercise habits and are critical in crafting a holistic view of someone's health status.

For instance, losing weight isn't going to help someone's health if they live in poverty, deal with discrimination in the workplace because of their gender identity, work three jobs, come home to a violent household, and have to live on four hours of sleep a night because of their work schedule. That being said, you can see that privilege plays a major role in health status, as it's easier for someone who is gender-conforming and in a higher social class to receive professional help to remove themselves from the violent relationship, find a higher paying nine-to-five job that requires a bachelor's degree, become a part of a welcoming, supportive community, and access a more balanced lifestyle.

Health shouldn't have to be a privilege, but in today's world, it unfortunately is.

Not only is the weight-normative approach marginalizing, it's also futile in terms of improving people's health. Doctors are tired of not seeing lasting results in patients who seek healthier lives, and so are patients. Medical professionals go into health care because they want to help people, and it's discouraging to continue to see people "fail" at losing weight to "improve" health. There's a better solution to this problem, and it's not as difficult or convoluted as we think.

Dr. Bacon and I discussed how the weight-normative framework in medicine and in our culture marginalizes people of color, gender identities, body sizes, and socioeconomic statuses. We discussed how HAES is the most sustainable way to instill behaviors that improve long-term health.

He noted:

"What we know is that weight is a poor proxy for everything that we've been told. . . . It doesn't measure good health, it doesn't measure one's eating habits, it doesn't measure one's exercise habits, it doesn't tell us anything about their character or background.

"I want to trash that old idea of using weight to help people and recognize the damage that we've done because we have used it in the past. And so, the new approach is to ask questions that are more direct that are really going to help people's lives. So, if we're interested in health behaviors, we can talk about them directly rather than making any kind of assumptions about weight."

Providers: Instead of assuming someone is unhealthy because of their appearance, ask direct questions on lifestyles and behaviors to open up a judgment-free conversation. It's impossible to understand someone's health status without having a working knowledge of their activity, nutrition, work life, home life, and mental health status. When the discussion becomes a two-way street, patients are much more likely to share information, which will allow you to be more helpful to them.

If a patient lives in a bigger body, they may have more particular needs. Patients who deal with weight stigma in their everyday lives are under more stress and will need coping skills to manage the discrimination they endure regularly. If a provider doesn't feel equipped to cover that, referring a patient to a therapist could be an alternative option.

Treating fat patients with compassion and kindness is the most important part of beginning to mend weight stigma in health care. If you're uncomfortable or have a negative attitude toward those in bigger bodies, ask yourself why.

Do you genuinely fear for their health, or have you internalized the messaging that weight equates to health in your studies and in your life without challenging it?

Would you feel shame if you looked like them?

Would you fear that people would pass judgments on you based on your size if you were fat?

If you do fear for their health status, what are the recommendations you'd make to that patient if they were thin?

Have an honest conversation with your patient.

"What are some ways we could take steps toward bettering your health?"

Maybe that's incorporating more fruits and veggies or going on a walk with a friend a few times a week. Maybe it's seeking help from a therapist to manage anxiety or depression or committing to a routine sleep schedule.

We know today that dieting and weight loss efforts haven't saved anyone, so why continue to try the same methods over and over again? If decades-long studies prove that weight loss isn't sustainable in the long run, why do we keep insisting that weight loss is the answer to our health issues? If we know that genetics, trauma, and social determinants of health play a larger role in body size than just food and exercise habits, why do we continue to blame people for their body size?

In science, studies are done to test whether a new method is better than the old one, and if the studies prove that the new finding is better, the old way gets thrown out, and the new one is adopted. Consider when people believed the Earth was at the center of the solar system hundreds of years ago. Scientists, mathematicians, and philosophers alike received pushback and were even accused of heresy for claiming that the Sun was at the center of our solar system. Eventually, however, people got on board, and now it's widely accepted that the Earth revolves around the Sun.

Dr. Bacon made a great comparison in our discussion that's worth sharing.

A few decades ago, being gay, lesbian, or bisexual was not accepted in society at all, and people believed that your gender and sexual orientation were a choice. You couldn't come out, you couldn't marry, and you were discriminated against for your sexuality. Now, although there's still more work to be done, it's becoming acceptable to openly identify as LGBTQ+.

Same-sex marriages are legal now, there's more representation in the media, and people in LGBTQ+ communities have more power than they did decades ago.

Right now, I believe we're in that midpoint in history where people still hold onto the old idea that dieting causes successful weight loss long-term, even though it's been proven for the past few decades that it doesn't work. We haven't gotten to the point where we've thrown that idea out the window. We can get there though, if we all work together to dismantle the fruitless promise of weight loss. Taking weight out of the conversation is a good start.

The idea that thinner is better is damaging to everyone, regardless of body size. Fat people are hurt the most by this narrative, and it's up to us to call out stigma when we see it and hold space for those who experience it. We weren't put on this Earth to shrink ourselves to fit the current trends or norms—we're here to share our experience and help others.

Dr. Bacon affirms that we must stop using weight as a marker for health if we're ever going to end weight stigma and throw out the myth of weight loss in health care. In the same way society once believed it was someone's "fault" they were queer, our society continues to perpetuate the harmful and false idea that it's someone's complete fault or choice that they're fat. If body size was so easy to manipulate, wouldn't everyone be thin to avoid the discrimination, shame, and stigma of being fat in today's world?

Dr. Bacon suggests that if you're a health care provider and have a fat client, ask yourself how you can support them to take care of their bodies. Nothing good comes out of hating or shaming ourselves into what our society considers "health."

Again, no one goes into health care with malicious intent. People go into health care to support and help others. If you're in health care and find yourself frustrated and at a loss as to how you can support your bigger clients, check out Health at Every Size. There are certifications available, but even reading Dr. Lindo Bacon's book, *Health At Every Size: The Surprising Truth About Your Weight,* will give you effective ways to support the improvement of patients' health without the old diet paradigms.

I recommend HAES to anyone who's struggled with their relationship with their bodies, and I hope that one day, we'll all look back and laugh at the silly notion that we can control our body's size and improve our health by shrinking it.

CHAPTER 11

WHY ALL DOCTORS SHOULD DITCH "WEIGHT MANAGEMENT" METHODS AND ADOPT INTUITIVE EATING AS HEALTH INTERVENTION

———

"There's a cartoon I just posted in my stories: it's only four little panes and it shows this person literally coming in with a detached arm. Their arm got severed, and they're sitting with their patient gown on, and they're like, 'Doctor, I have a problem with my arm,' and all the doctor sees is his fat body and says, 'Oh you just need to change your diet, you just need to lose weight—you'll feel a lot better.'"

Evelyn Tribole, MS, RDN, CEDRD-S, co-author of *Intuitive Eating: A Revolutionary Program That Works* with Elyse

Resch, MS, RD, FADA, summed up medical fatphobia in a nutshell by sharing this funny meme with me.

"When someone's in a larger body and they refuse to get weighed it's really, really a problem, and I've seen people strong armed over it."

One friend of Evelyn's got into a power struggle with the nurse practitioner over getting weighed until the practitioner told her she can't have the appointment.

"Now patients don't want to come in and have health care, and that's not good for health care either. Then there's underlying conditions going on and by the time they come, things have gotten worse. There's so many stories of this, so many stories."

Evelyn and I talked about flawed practices in medicine and in dieting. As an esteemed registered dietician that has taught thousands of people how to have a healthy relationship with food through her books, workbooks, workshops, and more, Evelyn has some great insight into why dieting doesn't work and what happens when we ban foods from our diet in the name of "health."

MYTH: One of the common fears people and medical professionals can have is that if we ditch the idea that we can lose weight by dieting, people will stop eating fruits and veggies completely and "lose control" over richer foods.

TRUTH: According to Evelyn Tribole, "Those types of fears usually come from a history of deprivation, and I hear common fears that 'I won't stop eating candy or chocolate or cookies or something,' and when you've had this deprivation both biologically and psychologically, it's often hard for that person to imagine that this could become ordinary, that food would still taste good."

It's the "paradox of permission," as she calls it.

What happens when we tell ourselves we can't have a certain food?

"Someone believes they can never have a food and they finally let themselves have it; they get to this last supper eating, and it's in this urgency and sometimes you aren't even tasting the food."

Sound familiar?

For me, I used to not be able to keep sweets in my house because I'd eat them all in one sitting. I had absolutely no control over foods that I deemed were "bad" or not a part of my "meal plan." It got to the point where I was so deprived of the foods I craved that I was eating my roommates' cookie dough, cereal, and cupcakes without their permission. It was a vicious cycle that caused me to be full of shame and guilt.

I never thought I'd be able to eat certain foods in normal amounts, but today, as I'm writing, I'm enjoying some candy that I've had in my pantry for the past three weeks and have been able to snack on here and there.

It took intervention by registered dietitians and professionals, along with a lot of trial and error, but the principles of intuitive eating taught me how to eat like a normal person again.

I had to give myself unconditional permission to eat *all* foods, not just the ones diet culture deemed "healthy."

Evelyn noted, "One of the things I noticed with people coming from diet culture is that there is a fair amount of dysregulation going on, where they don't know their body because they're so used to outsourcing it to other people."

In these cases, it may be necessary to start small, and work on some aspects of intuitive eating before going all in.

"It's easier to make peace with food when your body's not ravenous anymore," Evelyn said.

Amen to that. For me, I couldn't figure out how to "gain control" of my last suppers with foods until I was actually eating enough for my body daily. In order to stop binging, I had to stop restricting foods from my diet.

MYTH: Something that often gets misunderstood about intuitive eating studies and principles is that it only applies to fad diets, and if a medical professional is advising about dieting, that changes the outcomes.

TRUTH: All forms of dieting have the same outcomes—they don't work long-term. Evelyn mentioned that most of the weight studies have been under medical supervision, so it doesn't matter who is advising your diet; it won't work.

Whether it's a Pinterest ten-day cleanse or a lifestyle of "clean eating," both are diets that will lead to a loss of control over food, and a loss of touch with the body.

Diet culture has completely hijacked people's ability to connect with their bodies and listen to its needs.

Often times, when coming from diet culture, it takes time to reconnect with hunger cues, cravings, what feels good in the body, and what doesn't. Diet culture teaches us that we can't trust our bodies, when in reality, our bodies know best, and they're going to do whatever they can to get what they need.

The "shapeshifting" form of diet culture has warped our idea of what our relationship with food should look like.

MYTH: Keto, Intermittent Fasting, and "Clean Eating" are lifestyles, not diets.

TRUTH: They are all forms of dieting.

The complexity and ability of diet culture to shift to current trends has made it so challenging for people to realize what's good for them and what's not. Evelyn agreed, "It's so insidious and I think that's why people can go longer having an eating disorder and not realize it because so many disordered eating behaviors have been normalized because of diet culture."

The principles of intuitive eating are incredibly helpful for anyone looking to take back their relationship with food. Whether you're a medical provider who wants to refer your patients to a way to heal their food relationship or just a patient, Intuitive Eating is the anti-diet of all diets.

These are the ten principles of intuitive eating:

1. Reject the Diet Mentality
2. Honor Your Hunger
3. Make Peace with Food
4. Challenge the Food Police
5. Discover the Satisfaction Factor
6. Feel Your Fullness
7. Cope with Your Emotions with Kindness
8. Respect Your Body
9. Movement—Feel the Difference
10. Honor Your Health—Gentle Nutrition

If you feel like you're at your wits' end with your relationship with food, or you're a provider who has run out of ways to help patients in terms of offering diet advice, consider intuitive eating. Intuitive eating is associated with positive physical and mental outcomes, including lower risk for ob*y and eating disorders.[101] Intuitive eating has been linked to gratitude, which had a direct effect on body appreciation, lower social comparison, and higher self-worth.[102] Not only does it improve physical health, it impacts mental health and overall well-being! There have been volumes of studies done on intuitive eating, so if you're interested in learning more, pick up the book and check out studies at intuitiveeating.org.

---

[101] Intuitive Eating, "Studies: Intuitive Eating Studies," The Original Intuitive Eating Pros.

[102] Homan KJ and Tylka TL, "Development and Exploration of the Gratitude Model of Body Appreciation in Women," *Body Image*, 2018.

CHAPTER 12

WEIGHT MANAGEMENT HAS NO PLACE IN EVIDENCE-BASED CARE

———

In late 2017 and early 2018 I spent a few months in eating disorder treatment in Colorado. I decided to see a rheumatoid and osteoporosis doctor to see if there was anything else I could do to alleviate my Raynaud's syndrome, a rare (but not serious) disorder that narrows blood vessels in the fingers and toes and can cause my fingers and toes to swell up, especially when it's cold out. Part of it can be due to genetics, but mine was exacerbated by my eating disorder.

A nurse walked me to my exam room. "Dr. Robertson will be with you shortly."

I took a deep breath and sat on the table. I was nervous. There's something about being a younger woman and seeing a male doctor that gives me anxiety—anxiety of not being heard or taken seriously, which is apparently a very common sentiment after sharing this story with others. My eyes wandered around the room, reading posters and ads to make the wait time go by faster. I noticed that this office had screens that flashed different ads in each exam room. *How modern*, I thought. A red advertisement popped up that read: "LIGHT DINNER, 94 CALORIE SOUP" with a thorough run-down of nutrition facts and ingredients for the "meal." Ninety-four calories for a meal? I don't count calories anymore, but my dietician's snack recommendations for me are typically in the four-hundred-calorie ballpark, and those are my snacks. A purple advertisement popped up next: "MEAL REPLACEMENT SHAKE: 225 CALORIES" with a picture-perfect Instagram-worthy shake followed by the recipe and nutrition facts. *What is this?* I thought. I'm at a rheumatoid and osteoporosis office—since when are those extreme-diet hubs?

If I'm being honest, I felt pretty activated about the ads. I hadn't been out of eating disorder treatment that long, and with my newfound understanding of how diets don't work long-term, along with my sensitivity to how harmful advertisements like this can be to vulnerable people, I started to think about how I could approach this conversation with my doctor whenever he came in.

I heard a strong knock on the door and Dr. Robertson stepped in. I shared with him my concerns, and he gave some advice on managing my symptoms and offered to prescribe me medicine for it. After we finished discussing what I came in for, he asked, "Do you have any other questions?"

I paused. I had been stewing in frustration and fear of how this conversation could go. I mustered up the courage to ask him about the advertisements that had been blinking in my face for the past half hour.

"Yeah, I noticed these ads about meal replacement ideas. I know that you're probably not in control on what gets advertised in here, but I feel like this isn't an appropriate place for them. A large number of people with osteoporosis and circulation issues have a history of an eating disorder, or currently have one, so I feel like the ads can be triggering or damaging to people. Ninety-four calories seems pretty extreme for a dinner."

Dr. Robertson looked down and scoffed. "We have a much bigger problem with obesity here than we do with eating disorders. A lot of our patients are extremely obese."

Flushed and out of energy to say anything else, I decided nothing I would say would change his opinion, so I thanked him and checked out.

I wanted to say that people can be both malnourished and fat. That going on restrictive diets can cause life-long damage to our metabolisms and cause us to expend less energy and thus gain more weight back long-term. That going on diets that extreme will just exacerbate binge eating and cause a terrible cycle of restricting, binging, feeling shame, and doing it all over again the next day. But I said what I could that day and didn't feel like trying to explain that in a quick doctor's appointment.

I got home and did some research on how many nutrition courses are required in medical school. The general consensus was this: not nearly enough.

Did you know that only one out of five American medical schools require students to take a nutrition course?

Doctors are often on the front lines as the first professionals we go to for nutrition advice, even though medical schools in the US only offer an average of 19.6 hours of nutrition education, according to a 2010 report in *Academic Medicine*.[103]

Dr. Louise Metz, a medical professional who runs Mosaic Comprehensive Care in Chapel Hill, NC, agreed that nutrition is not addressed enough in medical school in an interview with Christy Harrison, MPH, RD, and CDN on Harrison's Food Psych podcast. When discussing the pressure doctors have to offer nutrition advice, Dr. Metz commented, "We are suddenly considered experts and we really are not. I think that my training was maybe a one- or two-hour online module during medical school."[104]

Dr. Metz had a unique approach in going into medicine, and her experiences shaped the way she practices medicine today. Let's look at how her practice has evolved, and how

---

[103] K.M. Adams, K.C. Lindell, M. Kohlmeier, S.H. Zeisel, "Status of Nutrition Education in Medical Schools," *Am J Clin Nutr.* 83 no. 4, (2006): 941S–944S.

[104] Christy Harrison, "Food Psych #207: Doctors Without Diet Culture with Louise Metz," September 30, 2019, in Food Psych Podcast, produced by Christy Harrison, Podcast, computer audio, 29:33.

she realized that weight management and body size talk had no place in evidence-based medicine.

Metz explained that her coursework in women's studies in biology at Duke University sparked her interest in the intersection of feminism and medical care.

"[I wanted] to approach medicine from a feminist perspective, and with an awareness of some of the problems with the standard paradigms in medicine, and really wanted to go into health care to try to help change things."[105]

Her early exposure to eating disorders in medical school paved the way for how she practices medicine today, but it took years of practicing to come to the conclusion that dieting did not fit in Dr. Metz's evidence-based practice. In Metz's third year of medical school, she had exposure to a patient with anorexia at a psychiatric inpatient facility who piqued her interest in eating disorders. She notes, "At the time, it wasn't something that was included in our training or our curriculum in med school at all. I had some friends . . . who are interested in this area, and we created a workshop to try to learn more about eating disorders. Also, as you may know, we don't learn much about nutrition as med students, so there was very little training at all on nutrition either."[106]

Later in medical school Metz was introduced to complexity theory by an internist she worked under who worked with eating disorders and also worked in women's health research.

---

[105] Ibid., 26:59.
[106] Ibid., 28:14.

Complexity theory involves analyzing systems that interact, so in medicine, that's looking at body systems that interact with each other and with the environment. This theory contrasted with western medicine's usual linear or reductive theories, where you look at a patient's problem list, separate things out, and don't look at how these separate problems can interact. This method stuck with Metz as she completed her residency in inner-city San Francisco, working with underserved patients. Weight was at the bottom of doctors' priority lists with those patients at the time. However, diet culture and weight management paradigms "crept in" when she began practicing with a more insured group of patients after medical school.

Dr. Metz remarked, "I think that just must have been ingrained from the parts that I had learned along the way in training, and then in society. Talking about weight management . . . was something I was doing then, but alongside that, I was taking care of patients with eating disorders, so there was definitely a really big contrast in what I was doing."[107]

When treating patients with eating disorders, there's a big focus on intuitive eating, letting go of the idea that body size can be controlled, blind weights or no weighing at all, and a larger focus on healthful behaviors, such as eating regular meals and snacks. Dr. Metz recalls having two completely different protocols for nurses when treating patients with eating disorders and patients without one:

"I thought I was practicing in a sort of non-diet way, because I was using terms like 'lifestyle changes,' or 'portion control,'

---

[107] Ibid., 31:19-36:17.

and of course, we know those are just different phrases for diet culture, but certainly looking back, I mean, the contrast was pretty stark in the work I was doing."[108]

So what caused Metz to ditch diet culture in treating patients?

Metz credits her sister, Anna Lutz, a registered dietician and eating disorder specialist, in opening her eyes to the Health at Every Size approach. Around the same time, Metz was looking to open her own practice.

Metz said, "I learned about a weight-inclusive approach. I was wanting to leave the bigger system where I was working because I really felt like it was hard for me to provide the type of care that I wanted to for my patients with all the constraints of a big system, so having to see patients in a fifteen-minute slot was very difficult. . . . I really felt like the system was not conducive to providing adequate and high-quality care, where we could really talk to our patients and provide holistic care."[109]

Metz now runs a practice that is rooted in the Health at Every Size approach, where she looks at patients holistically, only weighs patients if there is a valid need for it—such as pregnancy, certain medication dosages, or if the patient is a growing child—and does not prescribe weight loss as a line of treatment.

Metz had to navigate around the underlying assumption in health care that weight equates to health and dismantle those

---

[108] Ibid., 37:11.
[109] Ibid., 43:07.

assumptions: "We have pretty good evidence about the effects of weight stigma, and the negative effects of weight cycling (losing weight and gaining it back), and the fact that the BMI scale does not equate to health if we look at those numbers."

Both Metz and Harrison agree that the baseline assumption that weight equates to health was never really analyzed in their schooling, and no one challenged it. Metz notes, "There's so much focus on evidence-based medicine. . . . Then, on the other hand, we are providing this type of care, this weight management care that is completely not based on evidence. For instance, we know . . . that dieting is completely ineffective, and that up to 98 percent of individuals who lose weight will regain the weight, and two-thirds of those typically regain more. Really, there aren't any other treatments that we would prescribe in our field where we would want to prescribe a treatment that would fail in such a high percentage of cases, which is sort of baffling that we're so focused on the evidence, but we just have a blind spot in this area."[110]

If you're a medical professional who may be questioning how you can get reimbursed by insurance if you don't put a weight into the field, Metz notes that "it may be a misconception" that weights are required by insurance companies. Her practice doesn't put anything in the weight field, doesn't use IDC-10 codes for body size, and gets reimbursed for all patient visits. In fact, often times the reason many bigger systems claim that weights are required is due to quality programs that use weights as a quality measure, in which some providers and systems can receive bonuses or productivity pay

---

[110] Ibid., 54:20-57:28.

based on the tracking of patients' weights. In other words, tracking patients' weights increases profits. Dr. Metz has been asked by insurance companies to participate in weight tracking quality measures, but she and her practice choose not to participate.

As a patient, you are by law not required to step on the scale. You do not have to get weighed. If you need to, you can tell your provider to fill the weight field with "refused."

Most of the time, it's not a problem. Every now and then, however, it may look like this:

"Miss ___, come on back."

"Alright, take your shoes off, let's get your weight."

"I'm not getting weighed today."

"You have to get weighed,"

"I'm not getting prescribed medicine; I don't have to get weighed"

"Well honey, I have to get your weight!"

"By law, I don't have to get weighed. Write down that I refused."

That's it! It can be scary to go against the grain in a place where you normally haven't, but it will be worth it if your weight is something that bothers you or causes the conversations to sway into the weight loss territory at your appointment. Like I said, more often than not, a nurse will simply say, "Okay!" and move on.

Dr. Metz looks at practicing weight-inclusive medicine as compassionate care. She urges providers to ask, "Are we really providing compassionate care with this weight management approach?"[111] Metz attended the Academy of Eating Disorders Conference this past spring and heard something that really struck a chord in her. Rachel Millner held a talk on preparing clients with eating disorders for the trauma of going to the doctor.

Metz stated, "To think that people have to go to treatment to prepare themselves to come into the place where they're supposed to be partnering with health care providers in pursuing their health and wellness, I mean, it's just horrifying. There's clearly a serious problem with our system if that is the case, and I think it really is. Really, it is trauma in the medical system. Patients who are marginalized really can experience trauma when they go in to see the doctor due to the bias and stigma that exists."[112]

So for providers, how can we shift our practice in a weight-inclusive way?

Metz urges providers to do no harm. Sit down with your patients and talk about their experiences. Point out the weight stigma and talk to them about it. Give them space to talk about their experiences and desires to lose weight. Weight cycling

---

[111] Ibid., 54:20-58:46.

[112] Ibid., 54:20-1:00:12.

increases the risk of diabetes, hypertension, and other health complications. Thus, dieting is a treatment that causes harm.

In the same way that medications can get removed by the FDA because they were found to be harmful, we can remove weight loss as a line of treatment. I encourage anyone in health care to research the effects of weight cycling and weight stigma, as it's often the mediator between what we usually see: Obesity equals X, Y, and Z disease.

So, in what ways is weight stigma harmful in treatment?

We can look at one example Metz shared in her interview with Harrison, her experience with being diagnosed with PCOS, and compare it to what it's like to be diagnosed with it in a bigger body.

Dr. Metz was diagnosed with PCOS, or polycystic ovary syndrome, before going into medicine during her undergrad years, and explained that from her point of view as a doctor now, she received an entirely different diagnostic process than many women do today.

She shared that, "What's sort of interesting about it, looking back now, is that you know I mentioned I had a really extensive testing for these symptoms and what I see in my patients now who have PCOS is they often don't get that kind of work up. It's sort of assumed if they present with irregular periods and hirsutism (excessive body hair growth) and they live in a larger body that they have PCOS."[113]

---

[113] Ibid., 23:50.

Harrison remarked, "That's interesting, and the fact that you didn't live in a larger body made them take it more seriously maybe, or made them want to rule out other conditions."[114]

Metz agreed; the way she was tested for PCOS was different than what she hears from her patients in larger bodies. She noted, "The first thing that someone with PCOS is told if they live in a larger body is to lose weight, and that's often considered the primary treatment for their condition. That was not something that I was ever told to do as part of my treatment. . . . You take two different people with the exact same symptoms, and the work-up and treatment can be completely different just based on body size, which really makes no sense and is definitely not evidence-based."[115]

Often, we look at the short-term effects of weight loss in medicine without looking at the long-term complications of eventually gaining weight back. Weight cycling actually exacerbates insulin resistance, which can make PCOS symptoms worse and increase chances of developing type 2 diabetes and cardiovascular disease. Much like the chicken-before-the-egg argument, being fat isn't what's immediately causing these diseases; it's much more complicated than that. The impact of experiencing stigma, yo-yo dieting, trauma, and even socioeconomic status plays a role in the development of the diseases we all blame obesity for. If we can take the time to listen to our patients, understand them from a holistic perspective, and practice medicine in a compassionate way, we can treat people of all shapes and sizes with equal respect.

---

[114] Ibid., 24:34.
[115] Ibid., 25:51.

Rather than writing off patients and offering up a new diet for them to try, let's aim to hear them out. Practicing healthful behaviors improves health outcomes much more effectively than weight loss does.[116] Weight loss and inevitable regain causes many more health problems than it's worth. By approaching health care at a Health at Every Size Approach, we can offer compassionate, evidence-based care that allows patients to feel safe and share their experiences with providers. I highly recommend anyone going into medicine or practicing medicine to read Lindo Bacon's book *Health at Every Size*, which provides ample research and solutions to approaching health in an inclusive, intersectional way sans weight loss, and Christy Harrison's *Anti-Diet*, a groundbreaking book that challenges readers to reject diet culture and reclaim their lives, to learn more about the harmful consequences of dieting and how we can improve healthful behaviors at all body sizes.

---

[116] Jon Robison, "Health at Every Size: Toward a New Paradigm of Weight and Health," *MedGenMed: Medscape General Medicine*, 7, no. 3, (July 2005): 13, 12.

CHAPTER 13

STORIES FROM THE DOCTOR'S OFFICE: HOW THESE WOMEN ADVOCATED FOR THEMSELVES

———

"This diagnosis is most common in obese women of child-bearing age."

Elizabeth's shoulders slumped forward on the examination table, face blank, numb to what she had just heard. She had been diagnosed with intracranial hypertension, IIH, after a whirlwind of optic eye exams, ER trips, MRI scans, and a spinal tap all within the last twenty-four hours.

To Elizabeth, her doctor's rationale was all too familiar.

"It's nothing new to me to go to the doctor and be told that all of my ailments could be cured by losing weight. I classify this as 'lazy medicine' because in reality, many health problems are not caused by being overweight."

This wasn't the first time she'd been told her weight was the problem. In the past, Elizabeth had been told that a low-fat diet paired with exercise would cure her neck pain, which was caused by trauma. In another situation, her pelvic pain was blamed on her higher body weight, when she actually had endometriosis.

"This diagnosis is strictly due to your weight. This medication will help absorb the excess cerebral spinal fluid, and weight loss will help you decrease symptoms and hopefully prevent you from completely losing vision in your eye."

That's going to be difficult, Elizabeth thought. As a person in recovery from an eating disorder, dieting is equivalent to drinking as a recovering alcoholic. It never ends well.

Later that month, spinal fluid leakage from her recent IIH diagnoses caused her to have a terrible spinal headache. Doctors had punctured her lumbar in an earlier procedure, which resulted in a necessary blood transfusion of Elizabeth's own blood.

The anesthesiologist struggled to administer anesthesia.

"The problem is that I keep hitting bone because you're a big girl."

He refused to use the radiological equipment and bent Elizabeth over the gurney to administer. She shrieked in a room that was only divided by curtains.

In that moment, "the physical pain quickly turned to shame."

After Elizabeth got home that day, she turned to the internet to learn more about her new diagnosis.

Risk factors included high weight, and a few others. Elizabeth came across one risk factor that caught her eye: lithium carbonate can cause IIH.

"My symptoms began six months ago when I was put on lithium for bipolar depression," she said. She sat in shock.

"I told my doctors about my mental health disorders, but nobody asked if I had ever taken lithium."

Lithium is a medication very commonly used to treat bipolar disorders.

"I don't take it anymore, because I had some other side effects, so it wasn't on my current chart. They had no way of knowing I had taken it, but if they saw that I had a history of bipolar disorder, they should have asked me about it."[117]

Even though lithium is a psychiatric medication, other medical doctors need to have an awareness of medications and their potential side effects.

Cue Elizabeth's dubbed "lazy medicine" argument.

---

[117] Elizabeth Pidgeon, "It's 'Lazy Medicine' When Doctors Blame Everything on Your Weight," *The Mighty,* June 18, 2019.

* * *

Sophia Carter-Kahn and April Quioh, fat activists and writers, shared their experiences at the doctor in an episode of their podcast, *She's All Fat.*

April and Sophia dedicate themselves to fat-positive activism in order to help others advocate for themselves.

Sophia has experienced fatphobia at the doctor for most of her life, and as a result of "lazy medicine," wasn't diagnosed properly for her autoimmune diseases until she was in her late twenties.

"When I was five, I had a white blood cell test done for symptoms I was experiencing. The only note the doctor left with my mom was 'too big, less dessert.'

"All of my issues were exacerbated by not being diagnosed soon enough—I would tell my symptoms and doctors would say it's because I'm fat and eating too much; every health condition I had was blamed on my weight."

Sophia took matters into her own hands and did some research on her symptoms. She printed some things out and took her research to the doctor and got tests done and is now properly diagnosed with autoimmune and gastrointestinal issues.

TIP: If your doctor says they don't need to run a test on you after you ask, tell them to write that the doctor refused to run tests in your chart. Nine times out of ten, they'll run the test.

April grew up around hospitals and had learned more ways to advocate for herself because her mother was a nurse. As a woman of color, April's mom told her that she has to exaggerate her symptoms to get doctor's attention away from things being a "weight problem." A simple example of exaggerating symptoms would be rating a headache pain as an eight or nine, rather than an accurate six.

One of April's most ridiculous experiences of fatphobia in medical settings happened when she was on a school trip to Qatar.

"As soon as I landed, I felt sick. I had an ear infection and went straight to the campus office and asked for ear drops. The doctor said, 'You wouldn't have an ear infection if you weren't so fat.'"[118]

As if an ear infection is even remotely correlated to our bodies' size . . .

Sophia wrote an article for Yahoo that offers six ways you can advocate for yourself at the doctor's office if you live in a bigger body:[119]

1. Find a doctor you can trust.
- You can find HAES-aligned professionals on the Health at Every Size database online at haescommunity.com

---

[118] Sophia Carter-Kahn and April K. Quioh, "Episode 2.5: She's All Fat Goes to the Doctor," March 1, 2018 in *She's All Fat*, produced by Sophie Carter-Khan, podcast, MP3 audio.

[119] Sophia Carter-Kahn, "How to Advocate for Yourself at the Doctor as a Fat Person," *Yahoo! Life*, January 4, 2018.

2. Practice what you need to say prior to your appointment.
- Activist Regan Chastain created some awesome notecards you can print out and bring to the doctor's on her website, danceswithfat.org, with helpful phrases, questions, and even studies to refer doctors to when discussing problems. The blog post with the cards is called "What to Say at the Doctor's Office."

3. Bring a friend or partner for support.
- If you're anything like me and can get tongue-tied when someone of authority writes you off, bringing a friend to advocate can help.

4. Ask not to be weighed.
- You legally don't have to be weighed. If you absolutely need to for medication dosage or something pressing, face away from the scale and ask for them not to tell you before stepping on. Afterwards, ask them to keep your weight private from you, and ask the front desk to white out/delete your weight and BMI from your discharge packet.
- Side note: If you get pushback for refusing to be weighed, tell them to write "refuse" in your chart, or say that you aren't legally required to get weighed.

5. Keep the focus of discussion on the problem you came in with and ask what they'd recommend to a thin person.
- Redirect the conversation back to the problem. If the conversation turns to weight loss or dieting, ask what would be recommended as treatment for thin people.

6. You can always get a second opinion!

- It's your health care, and you have a right to ask for what you need. Seek a second opinion. If an office doesn't have medical equipment that suits your size, ask for somewhere that does. It's not your fault that they aren't equipped properly for people of all body types.[117]

* * *

You might think this stuff isn't that big of a deal. You may think, "Well, yeah, o*y is a problem, and people need to get told to lose weight for the sake of their health."

Or maybe you say, "These seem like isolated events, extreme ones for that matter."

If you're a medical provider, you may even be encouraged to promote weight loss to larger patients as something that will benefit their health.

As much as medical providers have been told to encourage weight loss for the benefit of patients' health, evidence has said the opposite. According to research, shaming people at the doctor's office actually does more harm than good.

Individuals who experience weight discrimination had a 60 percent higher mortality risk than people who didn't. Florida State University College of Medicine researchers examined data of over eighteen thousand individuals from several longitudinal studies that observed indicators of mortality risk: BMI, subjective health, disease burden, depressive symptoms, smoking history, and physical activity. It wasn't a higher BMI that increased mortality; it was weight discrimination.[120]

In another study of over three hundred autopsy reports, o*e patients were 1.65 times more likely to have a significant, undiagnosed medical condition than their thinner counterparts. People in bigger bodies are more likely to get misdiagnosed, if diagnosed at all, than people who are thinner and are more likely to have inadequate access to health care.

Thousands and thousands of people are walking around with undiagnosed health problems because they live in bigger bodies and were told their health issues were of their own making. Thousands of people are trying to lose weight to cure an issue that won't be fixed with weight loss.

In a symposium that tackled the subject of medical fatphobia, "Weapons of Mass Distraction—Confronting Sizeism," presenter Joan Chrisler, PhD, said that "recommending different treatments for patients with the same condition based on their weight is unethical and a form of malpractice," yet it's happening every day across the country.

"Research has shown that doctors repeatedly advise weight loss for fat patients while recommending CAT scans, blood work, or physical therapy for other, average weight patients."[121]

---

[120] Doug Carlson, "Weight Discrimination Linked to Increased Risk of Mortality," *Florida State University News*, October 15, 2015.

[121] American Psychological Association, "Fat Shaming in the Doctor's Office Can Be Mentally and Physically Harmful: Health Care Providers May Offer Weight Loss Advice in Place of Medical Treatment, Researchers Say," *ScienceDaily*, August 3, 2017.

Why is it that thinner patients are getting treatment plans that involve more testing, while larger patients are getting prescribed weight loss?

If weight discrimination is associated with an increased risk of dying, why does our society continue to do it?

Our fear of fatness (fatphobia) and beliefs that fat is bad and something we need to avoid at all costs is what keeps us in the cycle of discrimination, self-loathing, and projection of our own fears onto others. We've confused healthful behaviors with weight loss behaviors and can't seem to separate the two. Why do we equate fatness with mortality and thinness to health?

Research has shown that promoting healthful behaviors in the absence of weight loss improves health outcomes and is more sustainable in the long run. In a study of women with a higher BMI aged thirty to forty-five, women who were in a group that promoted health in a weight-neutral approach had greater improvements in intuitive eating and had larger reductions in LDL cholesterol than the weight loss group.[122]

The study measured metabolic fitness, including blood lipids and blood pressure, energy expenditure, eating behaviors, self-esteem, body image, and depression. The subjects who improved health behaviors without weight loss in mind established long-term behavioral changes that improved

---

[122] J.L. Mensinger, R.M. Calogero, S. Stranges, T.L. Tylka, "A Weight-Neutral versus Weight-Loss Approach for Health Promotion in Women with High BMI: A Randomized-Controlled Trial," *Appetite*. 105 (2016): 364–374.

health, while subjects who pursued weight loss did not. The weight was eventually regained in the dieting group, and health behaviors were not sustained.[123]

Maybe you're a parent and you fear that your child is getting chubby and don't want him to be bullied at school, so you try to control his food intake or sign him up for more activities. Or maybe your older brother has gained weight, and you repeatedly try to get him to join a gym or go on a diet. Although there's nothing inherently wrong with wanting to promote eating nutritious food or exercising to loved ones, it's the messages underneath that are harmful and fatphobic when suggested as part of changing one's body.

This is not to say that eating nutrient-dense foods or exercising is fatphobic; it's not. What's fatphobic is to assume that someone is fat solely because of their own personal eating and exercise habits. Elizabeth, April, and Sophia all experienced weight bias at the doctor when their health problems had nothing to do with their weight.

What's worse is that not only is fatphobia keeping people from accessing proper care, it's harming people's mental health. No one should have to experience teasing and belittling comments in the medical space. Every person should be treated with equal respect, no matter their appearance or pant size.

There's a way to promote healthful behaviors without weight loss or body discrimination being a part of the equation, but

---

[123] Bacon, Linda et al., "Size Acceptance and Intuitive Eating Improve Health for Obese, Female Chronic Dieters," *Journal of the American Dietetic Association* 105, no. 6 (2005): 929–36.

we've associated so much of health with weight loss that it's difficult for many to separate the two. If the way that we promote health is getting in the way of our mental health or physical health, we have a problem. The solution to that is taking weight loss out of the prescription.

If you experience fatphobia in medical care, take Sophia's advice and prepare for your visit. Bring a friend, practice what you need to say, ask for testing, do your research, and refuse to get weighed unless it's necessary for proper medication dosage. Take power back into your own hands, and if a doctor denies running a test, ask for them to write that in your chart. Chances are, they'll run the test.

It's not right that you have to deal with discrimination, but it is your right to receive adequate health care, and you can with the right actions.

CONCLUSION

Society has chosen to ignore and even encourage one of the most normalized forms of discrimination today.

Fatphobia is killing people. Whether it be misdiagnoses or altogether health care avoidance, fat people aren't getting the same level of care that thinner people are, and the inherent bias in our medical system is causing providers to miss vital diagnoses.

Fatphobia is impacting people's mental health, physical health, pay, insurance, and overall quality of life and mortality.

We were all born into a world that grooms society to favor a "palatable" appearance that suits the current body ideal. That is not our fault.

It's one thing for a society to have preferences or norms (whether they are positive or negative), but when that preference crosses into a territory where it's interfering with people's medical care and life, it's clearly gone too far.

This is what has happened in the United States, and in several other countries around the world.

Fatphobia, weight bias, size discrimination, whatever you want to call it, is harming people each and every day. It's impacting physical and mental health, and in some cases, like we saw in Jan's story, it's killing people. Doctors are missing critical diagnoses because of assumptions made based upon a patient's body size.

Everybody has a right to receive the same level of treatment as the next person, regardless of how they look.

Yes, it's ingrained into our culture.

Yes, it's embedded into frameworks of our health systems.

It's all over television, social media, workspaces, and classrooms.

But: We don't have to continue to live in that narrative if we don't want to.

We are all responsible to ensure that the next generation is treated equally in health care and in life, whether they be fat, skinny, black, or brown.

Start the conversations. Share books. Share your stories. Speak up.

Now is the time to become a catalyst for change, whether you're a patient who's ready to advocate for yourself, you're a doctor who's frustrated with the futility of diet advice, you're a student looking into a career path in health care, or you're an activist by night, worker by day.

If you're a medical professional and you're ready to advocate and treat your fat patients as you would a thin patient, you can be that person who positively impacts someone's experience in the doctor's office forever.

You can give that life-changing diagnosis that can be treated early before it's too late.

You can be the advocate who helps other professionals break down their own fatphobia.

If you're a patient, use the resources in this book. Find a HAES-aligned doctor in your area or bring these principles into your appointment, refuse to be weighed, advocate for yourself, or bring a friend for support. You deserve compassionate care. Help your friends in their journey in taking their power back at the doctor's office.

This isn't an overnight job—but it's worth the fight.

In the world of science, we're always throwing out antiquated practices once new information and new studies prove better solutions. If we didn't, we'd still be bloodletting and throwing leeches on people to cure illness like we did in the Middle Ages.

We've failed to improve health outcomes by insisting that thinness is health. In fact, we've made health outcomes worse.

By upholding fatphobia, consciously or subconsciously, our medical system and our culture has increased mental distress and negatively impacted mental health, increased rates of disordered eating and eating disorders, increased health care avoidance, and has caused many people to not receive the diagnoses they need to improve their health.

People are dying because our society values size and appearance more than anything. It's up to us to ensure that we don't allow this to continue.

If providers, health professionals, and people alike can find it in their hearts to see past body size, we can all work toward making health care more just. The basic human rights of fat people shouldn't even be up for debate.

It's time to toss out the old paradigm that losing weight is going to solve all of our problems; we have known for decades that it doesn't work.

Let's analyze each individual's medical concerns without a side of fatphobia. We are all so much more whole and complex than that.

APPENDIX

INTRODUCTION

Begley, Sharon. "Insight: America's Hatred of Fat Hurts Obesity Fight," *Health News: Reuters* (article), May 11, 2012. https://www.reuters.com/article/us-obesity-stigma/insight-americas-hatred-of-fat-hurts-obesity-fight-idUSBRE84A0PA20120511.

Centers for Disease Control and Prevention (CDC). "Obesity and Overweight." National Center for Health Statistics. Last Reviewed February 28, 2020. https://www.cdc.gov/nchs/fastats/obesity-overweight.htm.

Cohen, Elizabeth and McDermott, Anne. "Who's Fat? New Definition Adopted," *CNN* (article), June 17, 1998. http://www.cnn.com/HEALTH/9806/17/weight.guidelines/.

Kindelan, Katie and M.Ginsburg, Jordena. "Woman Says She Was Told by Her Doctor to Lose Weight. Then She Discovered It Was Cancer," *Good Morning America* (article), August 16, 2019. https://www.goodmorningamerica.com/wellness/story/woman-told-doctor-lose-weight-discovered-cancer-65010413.

LaRosa, John. "Top 9 Things to Know About the Weight Loss Industry," *Market Research Blog,* March 6, 2019. https://blog.marketresearch.com/u.s.-weight-loss-industry-grows-to-72-billion.

Puhl, R., Andreyeva, T. and Brownell, K. "Perceptions of Weight Discrimination: Prevalence and Comparison to Race and Gender Discrimination in America." *Int J Obes* 32, 992–1000 (2008). https://doi.org/10.1038/ijo.2008.22.

Walden, Foster, Letizia, Stunkard, "A Multicenter Evaluation of a Proprietary Weight Reduction Program for the Treatment of Marked Obesity." Deception and Fraud in The Diet Industry, Part IV Hearing, 102 no. 78 (May 1992): 961. https://books.google.com/books?id=YBtkDVyyqioC&pg=PA180&lpg=PA180&dq=how+much+was+the+diet+industry+worth+in+1990&source=bl&ots=5Y7oqDhL4h&sig=ACfU3U1YyZiZE9JogQ-P7FTbLwq95uzB2Q&hl=en&sa=X&ved=2ahUKEwiUl7qGw7noAhVqQt-8KHcARCC8Q6AEwDHoECAoQAQ#v=onepage&q=how%20much%20was%20the%20diet%20industry%20worth%20in%201990&f=false.

CHAPTER 1: DIET CULTURE'S HEAVY HAND

A. Ferdman, Roberto. "Why Diets Don't Actually Work, According to a Researcher Who Has Studied Them for Decades." *Washington Post: Economic Policy,* May 4, 2015. https://www.washingtonpost.com/news/wonk/wp/2015/05/04/why-diets-dont-actually-work-according-to-a-researcher-who-has-studied-them-for-decades/.

Crowe, Kelly. "Obesity Research Confirms Long-Term Weight Loss Almost Impossible." *CBC News,* June 4, 2014. https://www.cbc.ca/news/health/obesity-research-confirms-long-term-weight-loss-almost-impossible-1.2663585.

Ducharme, Jamie. "About Half of Americans Say They're Trying to Lose Weight." *Time,* July 12, 2018. https://time.com/5334532/weight-loss-americans/.

Dulloo, Abdul G., Jean Jacquet, and Jean-Pierre Montani. "How Dieting Makes Some Fatter: From a Perspective of Human Body

Composition Autoregulation." *Proceedings of the Nutrition Society* 71, no. 3 (2012): 379–89. doi:10.1017/S0029665112000225.

Durkin, Mollie. "Doctor, Your Weight Bias Is Showing." *ACP Internist Conference Coverage,* February 2017. https://acpinternist. org/archives/2017/02/weight.htm.

Fruh, S. M., Nadglowski, J., Hall, H. R., Davis, S. L., Crook, E. D., and Zlomke, K. "Obesity Stigma and Bias." *The Journal for Nurse Practitioner : JNP,* 12(7) (2016), 425–432. https://doi.org/10.1016/j. nurpra.2016.05.013.

Harrison, Christy. "What Is Diet Culture?" *Christy Harrison* (blog), August 0, 2018. https://christyharrison.com/blog/what-is-diet-culture#:~:text=Diet%20culture%20is%20a%20system,the%20 impossibly%20thin%20%E2%80%9Cideal.%E2%80%9D.

M. Shisslak, Catherine, PhD, Crago, Marjorie, PhD, and S. Estes, Linda, PhD. "The Spectrum of Eating Disturbances." *The International Journal of Eating Disorders* (November 1995). https://doi.org/10.1002/1098-108X(199511)18:3<209::AID-EAT2260180303>3.0.CO;2-E.

Rothblum, E. D. "Slim Chance for Permanent Weight Loss." *Archives of Scientific Psychology,* 6(1), 63–69. http://dx.doi.org/10.1037/ arc0000043.

Wallis, Lucy. "Do Slimming Clubs Work?" *BBC News,* August 8, 2013. https://www.bbc.com/news/magazine-23463006.

Wolpert, Stuart. "Dieting Does Not Work, UCLA Researchers Report." *UCLA Newsroom: Science and Technology,* April 3, 2007. https://newsroom.ucla.edu/releases/Dieting-Does-Not-Work-UCLA-Researchers-7832.

CHAPTER 2: RACISM, FATPHOBIA, AND ITS IMPACT ON THE "O WORD" EPIDEMIC

"The Five Solas." *Introduction to Protestantism.* Accessed April 2020, http://protestantism.co.uk/solas.

Brumberg, Fasting Girls, 231.

CDC. "Obesity Epidemic Increases Dramatically in the United States: CDC Director Calls for National Prevention Effort." Last Modified October 26, 1999. https://www.cdc.gov/media/pressrel/r991026.htm#:~:text=Obesity%20.

Cigna. "Health Disparities: African-American or Black Population." Last Modified April 2016. https://www.cigna.com/static/www-cigna-com/docs/health-care-providers/african-american-health-disparities.pdf.

Czerniawski, Amanda M. "From Average to Ideal: The Evolution of the Height and Weight Table in the United States, 1836–1943." Social Science History 31, no. 2 (2007): 273–96. Accessed September 10, 2020. doi:10.2307/40267940.

Flegal et al., "Prevalence and Trends in Obesity among US Adults."

Forth, Christopher. "Fat, Desire and Disgust in the Colonial Imagination," History Workshop Journal 73, no. 1 (2012): 214.

Frieden, Joyce. "Action Needed to Cut Disparities in Black Maternal, Child Mortality." Medpage Today, December 12, 2018. https://www.medpagetoday.com/obgyn/pregnancy/76882.

John V. Gaff, "Obesity as a Cause of Sterility," Journal of the American Medical Association 28, no. 4 (Jan. 23, 1897): 166–68.

Katherine M. Flegal, Brian K. Kit, Heather Orpana, and Barry I. Graubard, "Association of All-Cause Mortality with Overweight and Obesity Using Standard Body Mass Index Categories: A Systematic Review and Meta-Analysis," Journal of the American Medical Association 309, no. 1 (2012): 71–82.

Kellogg, Ladies' Guide in Health and Disease, 392.

Kellogg, Ladies' Guide in Health and Disease, 169.

Kelly M. Hoffman, Sophie Trawalter, Jordan R. Axt, and M. Norman Oliver. "Racial Bias in Pain Assessment and Treatment Recommendations, and False Beliefs about Biological Differences between Blacks and Whites." *PNAS* April 19, 2016 113 (16) 4296–4301; first published April 4, 2016; https://doi.org/10.1073/pnas.1516047113.

Leigh Hunt, "Chapter on Female Features," *Godey's Lady's Book*, April 1836.

M. Tester, June, Tess C. Lang, and Barbara A. Laraia. "Disordered Eating Behaviours and Food Insecurity: A Qualitative Study about Children with Obesity in Low-Income Households." *Obesity Research & Clinical Practice*, 10, no. 5, (September–October 2016): 544–552. https://doi.org/10.1016/j.orcp.2015.11.007.

Minter, Marc. "Luther & the 'Five Solas' of the Reformation," *Wordpress* (blog), April 12, 2014. https://marcminter.com/2014/04/12/luther-the-five-solas-of-the-reformation/.

Moffet, Thomas, Christopher Bennet, and Thomas Osborne. *Health's Improvement, or, Rules comprizing and discovering the nature, method and manner of preparing all sorts of foods used in this nation [...] corrected and enlarged by Christopher Bennet ... to which is now prefix'd A Short view of the Author's Life and Writings, by Mr. Oldys. And an introduction, by R. James, M.D.* London: Printed for T. Osborne, in Gray's Inn, 1746.

Mozes, Alan. "Underweight Even Deadlier Than Overweight, Study Says," *WebMD*, last modified March 28, 2014, https://www.webmd.com/diet/news/20140328/underweight-even-deadlier-than-overweight-study-says.

Nuttall F. Q. (2015). Body Mass Index: Obesity, BMI, and Health: A Critical Review. *Nutrition today, 50*(3), 117–128. https://doi.org/10.1097/NT.0000000000000092.

Peabody, Sue. *There Are No Slaves in France* (Oxford Scholarship Online: October 2011).

Purchas, Samuel. *Hakluytus Posthumus or, Purchas His Pilgrimes: Contayning a History of the World in Sea Voyages and Lande Travells by Englishmen and Others.* Vol. 16. Cambridge Library Collection—Maritime Exploration. Cambridge: Cambridge University Press, 2014, doi: 10.1017/CBO9781316050699.

Salimah H. Meghani, PhD, MBE, Eeeseung Byun, PhD(c), Rollin M. Gallagher, MD, MPH, "Time to Take Stock: A Meta-Analysis and Systematic Review of Analgesic Treatment Disparities for Pain in the United States," *Pain Medicine*, Volume 13, Issue 2, February 2012, Pages 150–174, https://doi.org/10.1111/j.1526-4637.2011.01310.x.

Stern, Alexandra Minna. "That Time the United States Sterilized 60,000 of Its Citizens." *HuffPost*, January 7, 2016. https://www.huffpost.com/entry/sterilization-united-states_n_568f35f2e-4b0c8beacf68713.

Strings, Sabrina. *Fearing the Black Body: The Racial Origins of Fat Phobia*. New York: NYU Press, 2019, 82–89.

University of Southern California. "Black Girls Are 50 Percent More Likely to Be Bulimic Than White Girls." ScienceDaily. www.sciencedaily.com/releases/2009/03/090318140532.htm.

Wilson, Dr. John Harvey Kellogg, 214.

Your Fat Friend. "The Bizarre and Racist History of the BMI," *Elemental.Medium* (blog) October 15, 2019. https://elemental.medium.com/the-bizarre-and-racist-history-of-the-bmi-7d8dc2aa33bb?.

CHAPTER 3: WHY WEIGHT LOSS ISN'T SUSTAINABLE: BIGGEST LOSER STUDY

Brink, Susan. "What Happens to The Body and Mind When Starvation Sets In?" *NPR (blog),* January 20, 2016. https://wamu.org/story/16/01/20/what_happens_to_the_body_and_mind_when_starvation_sets_in/.

Callahan, Maureen. "The Brutal Secrets Behind *The Biggest Loser.*" *New York Post: Entertainment,* January 18, 2015. https://nypost.com/2015/01/18/contestant-reveals-the-brutal-secrets-of-the-biggest-loser/.

Fothergill, E., Guo, J., Howard, L., Kerns, J.C., Knuth, N.D., Brychta, R., Chen, K.Y., Skarulis, M.C., Walter, M., Walter, P.J. and Hall, K.D. "Persistent Metabolic Adaptation 6 Years After *The Biggest Loser* Competition." *Obesity,* 24, (2016): 1612–1619. doi:10.1002/oby.21538.

"Is Sudden Weight Loss Causing Hair Loss?" *Business Standard: Health Medical Pharma,* updated April 23, 2018. https://www.business-standard.com/article/news-ians/is-sudden-weight-loss-causing-hair-loss-118042300866_1.html#:~:text=*%20Hair%20loss%20after%20weight%20loss,weight%20loss%20must%20be%20gradual.

"Stopped or Missed Periods." *NHS,* last reviewed August 2, 2019. https://www.nhs.uk/conditions/stopped-or-missed-periods/.

Kolata, Gina. "After *The Biggest Loser,* Their Bodies Fought to Regain Weight." *New York Times,* May 2, 2016. https://www.nytimes.com/2016/05/02/health/biggest-loser-weight-loss.html.

Wolpert, Stuart. "Dieting Does Not Work, UCLA Researchers Report." *UCLA Newsroom: Science and Technology,* April 3, 2007. https://newsroom.ucla.edu/releases/Dieting-Does-Not-Work-UCLA-Researchers-7832.

CHAPTER 4: FATPHOBIA AND HEALTHCARE AVOIDANCE

Forhan, Mary, Salas, Ximena Ramos. "Inequities in Healthcare: A Review of Bias and Discrimination in Obesity Treatment." *Canadian Journal of Diabetes 37,* no. 3 (June 2013): 205-209. https://doi.org/10.1016/j.jcjd.2013.03.362.

Phelan, S.M., Dovidio, J.F., Puhl, R.M., Burgess, D.J., Nelson, D.B., Yeazel, M.W., Hardeman, R., Perry, S. and van Ryn, M. "Implicit and Explicit Weight Bias in a National Sample of 4,732 Medical Students: The Medical Student CHANGES Study." *Obesity,* 22, (2014): 1201–1208. doi:10.1002/oby.20687.

Poon, M.-Y. and Tarrant, M. "Obesity: Attitudes of Undergraduate Student Nurses and Registered Nurses." *Journal of Clinical Nursing,* 18, (2009): 2355-2365. doi:10.1111/j.1365-2702.2008.02709.x.

Puhl R.M., Heuer C.A. "Obesity StigmA: Important Considerations for Public Health." *Am J Public Health*. 2010;100(6):1019–1028. doi:10.2105/AJPH.2009.159491.

Visit https://implicit.harvard.edu/implicit/selectatest.html. to take the implicit weight bias test.

Whitfield, Kenyetta. "Fat, Black Women's Bodies Are Under Attack. Why Did It Take a Thin White Man to Get Our Cries Heard?" *Rewire News,* October 12, 2018. https://rewire.news/article/2018/10/12/fat-black-womens-bodies-are-under-attack-why-did-it-take-a-thin-white-man-to-get-our-cries-heard/.

" Why Are Black Women at Such High Risk of Dying from Pregnancy Complications?"*America Heart Association News,* February 20, 2019. https://www.heart.org/en/news/2019/02/20/why-are-black-women-at-such-high-risk-of-dying-from-pregnancy-complications.

Wu, Y. and Berry D. "Impact of Weight Stigma on Physiological and Psychological Health Outcomes for Overweight and Obese Adults: A Systematic Review." *J Adv Nurs*. (2017): 1–13.

Your Fat Friend. "Weight Stigma Kept Me Out of Doctors' Offices for Almost a Decade." *Self,* June 26, 2018. https://www.self.com/story/weight-stigma-kept-me-out-of-doctors-offices.

CHAPTER 5: FATPHOBIA AND LATE DIAGNOSES

Alberga, Angela S. et al. "Weight Bias and Health Care Utilization: A Scoping Review." *Primary Health Care research & Development* 20, no. 116, (July 2019): doi: 10.1017/S1463423619000227.

Carlson, Doug. "Weight Discrimination Linked to Increased Risk of Mortality." *Florida State University News,* October 15, 2015. https://news.fsu.edu/news/health-medicine/2015/10/15/weight-discrimination-linked-to-increased-risk-of-mortality/.

Fraser, Laura. "My Sister's Cancer Might Have Been Diagnosed Sooner—If Doctors Could Have Seen beyond Her Weight." *Stat* (blog), August 15, 2017. https://www.statnews.com/2017/08/15/cancer-diagnosis-weight-doctors/.

Kindelan, Katie and M. Ginsburg, Jordena. "Woman Says She Was Told by Her Doctor to Lose Weight. Then She Discovered It Was Cancer," *Good Morning America* (article), August 16, 2019. https://www.goodmorningamerica.com/wellness/story/woman-told-doctor-lose-weight-discovered-cancer-65010413.

Okwerekwu, Jennifer Adaze. "In treating obese patients, too often doctors can't see past weight." *Stat* (blog), June 3, 2016. https://www.statnews.com/2016/06/03/weight-obese-doctors-patients/.

CHAPTER 6: EMPLOYERS, INSURANCE COVERAGE, AND FATPHOBIA

Ahmed-Haq, Rubina. "Fatphobia in the Workplace Can Be Career Limiting and Psychologically Harmful." *CBC News,* November 1, 2018. https://www.cbc.ca/news/canada/fatphobia-in-the-workplace-can-be-career-limiting-and-psychologically-harmful-1.4878398.

Anonymous. "Punitive Wellness Programs Are Already Here." *ConscienHealth* (blog), April 4, 2013. https://conscienhealth.org/2013/04/punitive-wellness-programs-are-here/.

Ellin, Abby. "How Obamacare Allows Companies to Punish Fat Employees." *Observer,* September 16, 2015. https://observer.com/2015/09/unwell-how-the-affordable-care-act-lets-companies-punish-fat-employees/.

Fontinelle, Amy. "How Much Does Health Insurance Cost?" *Investopedia,* last updated Oct 28, 2019. https://www.investopedia.com/articles/personal-finance/030116/why-higher-bmi-shouldnt-raise-insurance-rates.asp.

Jackson, Cedric. "How Does Health Insurance for Obese People Work?" *Freeway Insurance,* March 13, 2020. https://www.freeway-insurance.com/knowledge-center/health-insurance/understanding-health-insurance/health-insurance-for-obese-people/#:~:text=How%20Can%20Obesity%20Increase%20Insurance,changed%20 the%20health%20insurance%20industry.&text=In%20some%20cases%2C%20health%20insurance,with%20a%20BMI%20below%2030.

Kinzel, Lesley. "New Study Finds That Weight Discrimination in the Workplace is Just as Horrible and Depressing as Ever." *Time,* November 28, 2014. https://time.com/3606031/weight-discrimination-workplace/.

O'Neill, Michael. "Fatphobia: America's Overlooked Form of Discrimination." *Brown Political Review,* October 10, 2016. https://brownpoliticalreview.org/2016/10/fatphobia-americas-overlooked-form-discrimination/.

Ortega, Francisco B et al. "The intriguing metabolically healthy but obese phenotype: cardiovascular prognosis and role of fitness." *European heart journal* vol. 34 no. 5 (2013): 389-97. doi:10.1093/ eurheartj/ehs174.

Shinall, Jennifer Bennett. "Occupational Characteristics and the Obesity Wage Penalty," *Vanderbilt Law and Economics Research Paper* no. 16–12 (October 7, 2015), Vanderbilt Public Law Research Paper No. 16–23, http://dx.doi.org/10.2139/ssrn.2379575.

Stateside Staff. "The Political Pioneer Who Gave Michigan's Civil Rights Law Its Name." *Michigan Radio* (website), March 10, 2020. https://www.michiganradio.org/post/political-pioneer-whogave-michigans-civil-rights-law-its-name.

"The Surprisingly Personal Health Questions Your Employer Can Ask You." *Money,* November 19, 2014. https://money.com/ health-risk-assessment-questionnaire/.

CHAPTER 7: FATPHOBIA AND QUACK DOCTORS

Berry, Ken D. Youtube Bio, written on October 8, 2017, https:// www.youtube.com/watch?v=qSEueWHLfLo.

Kalayjian, Tro. "200 years ago, before refrigerators, microwaves & Uber Eats; "time-restricted feeding" was "eating," "Whole food plant based" was "summer/autumn," "Keto/carnivore" was "winter/spring," "Alternate day fasting" was "it got away," Yet, dietitians call them eating disorders," Twitter, March 12, 2020. https://twitter.com/rhythmnutrition/status/1238794958896857088.

Kaplan, Karen. "Real-World Doctors Fact-Check Dr. Oz, and the Results Aren't Pretty." *LA Times,* December 19, 2014. https://www.latimes.com/science/sciencenow/la-sci-sn-dr-oz-claims-fact-check-bmj-20141219-story.html.

Schein, Michael. "Dr. Oz Makes Millions Even Though He's Been Called a 'Charlatan' (And You Should Follow His Lead)." *Forbes,* May 25, 2018. https://www.forbes.com/sites/michaelschein/2018/05/25/dr-oz-makes-millions-even-though-hes-a-total-fraud-and-other-reasons-you-should-follow-his-lead/#38ba57645fe1.

Specter, Michael. "The Operator: Is the Most Trusted Doctor in America Doing More Harm Than Good?" *New Yorker,* January 28, 2013. https://www.newyorker.com/magazine/2013/02/04/the-operator?currentPage=all.

Tilburt, Jon C., Megan Allyse, and Frederic W. Hafferty. "The Case of Dr. Oz: Ethics, Evidence, and Does Professional Self-Regulation Work?" *AMA J Ethics,* 19 no. 2 (2017):199–206. doi: 10.1001/journalofethics.2017.19.2.msoc1-1702.

CHAPTER 8: CHILDREN AND FATPHOBIA

"Statistics About Diabetes." *American Diabetes Association.* Accessed April 17, 2020, https://www.diabetes.org/resources/statistics/statistics-about-diabetes.

Bacon, L., & Aphramor, L. *Body Respect: What Conventional Health Books Get Wrong, Leave Out, and Just Plain Fail to Understand about Weight.* Dallas: BenBella Books, 2014.

"Facts About Child Hunger in America." *No Kid Hungry,* Accessed April 18, 2020, https://www.nokidhungry.org/who-we-are/hunger-facts.

"Mid-year Population by Youth Age Groups and Sex - Custom Region - United States." *United States Census: International Programs.* Accessed April 17, 2020, https://www.census.gov/data-tools/demo/idb/region.php?T=4&RT=0&A=both&Y=2014&C=US&R=.

Peeke, Pamela. "Just What IS an Average Woman's Size Anymore?" *WebMD,* January 25, 2010. https://blogs.webmd.com/from-our-archives/20100125/just-what-is-an-average-womans-size-anymore.

Slattengren, Kathy. "Publicly or Privately Shaming Harms Kids." *Priceless Parenting* (blog), Accessed April 18, 2020, https://www.pricelessparenting.com/documents/shaming-harms-kids.

STRIPED. "Report: Economic Costs of Eating Disorders." Harvard T.H. Chan School of Public Health (June 2020). https://www.hsph.harvard.edu/striped/report-economic-costs-of-eating-disorders/.

Stunkard, A. and McLaren-Hume, M. "The Results of Treatment for Obesity: A Review of the Literature and Report of a Series." *AMA Arch Intern Med.* (1959);103(1):79–85. doi:10.1001/archinte.1959.00270010085011.

CHAPTER 9: THE DANGERS OF GASTRIC BYPASS SURGERY

"Bariatric Surgery." *Mayo Clinic,* January 22, 2020. https://www.mayoclinic.org/tests-procedures/bariatric-surgery/about/pac-20394258.

"Information on Bariatric Surgery." *US News & World Report,* Last Reviewed January 8, 2010. https://health.usnews.com/health-conditions/heart-health/information-on-bariatric-surgery/overview.

Hamilton, Amber. "New Study Finds Most Bariatric Surgeries Performed in Northeast, and Fewest in South Where Obesity Rates are Highest, and Economies are Weakest." *American Society for Metabolic and Bariatric Surgery,* November 15, 2018. https://asmbs.org/articles/new-study-finds-most-bariatric-surgeries-performed-in-northeast-and-fewest-in-south-where-obesity-rates-are-highest-and-economies-are-weakest#:~:text=In%202017%2C%20228%2C000%20bariatric%20procedures,least%2040%20(severe%20obesity).

Landsverk, Gabby. "A Woman Died of Malnutrition after Weight-Loss Surgery Led Her Lose 250 Pounds over 10 Years." *Insider,* October 18, 2019. https://www.insider.com/woman-died-weight-loss-surgery-bariatric-surgery-risks-2019-10.

Logue, Katie. "When Gastric Bypass Surgery Goes Horribly Wrong." *Her View from Home* (blog), Accessed May 8, 2020. https://herviewfromhome.com/when-gastric-bypass-surgery-goes-horribly-wrong/.

Morales, Tatiana. "Gastric Bypass Surgery Gone Bad." *CBS News,* January 21, 2005. https://www.cbsnews.com/news/gastric-bypass-surgery-gone-bad/.

Siegfried, Donna. "Rates of Drug-, Alcohol-Linked Death Triple After Weight Loss Surgery." *US News,* June 20, 2019. https://www.usnews.com/news/health-news/articles/2019-06-20/rates-of-drug-alcohol-linked-death-triple-after-weight-loss-surgery.

CHAPTER 10: HAES AND WHY IT WORKS

"HAES includes the following basic components:" *HAES Community,* last reviewed 2020. https://haescommunity.com/.

"HAES® Principles." *ASDAH: Association for Size Diversity and Health,* last reviewed 2020. https://www.sizediversityandhealth.org/content.asp?id=76.

CHAPTER 11: WHY ALL DOCTORS SHOULD DITCH "WEIGHT MANAGEMENT" METHODS AND ADOPT INTUITIVE EATING AS HEALTH INTERVENTION

"Homan KJ and Tylka TL. (2018). "Development and Exploration of the Gratitude Model of Body Appreciation in Women." *Body Image.* 2018 Feb 8;25:14–22. doi: 10.1016/j.bodyim.2018.01.008.

"Intuitive Eating. "Studies: Intuitive Eating Studies." The Original Intuitive Eating Pros. website. 2007–2019. https://www.intuitiveeating.org/resources/studies/#:~:text=Intuitive%20eating%20is%20an%20adaptive,and%20eating%20disorders%20(EDs).

CHAPTER 12: STORIES FROM THE DOCTOR'S OFFICE: HOW THESE WOMEN ADVOCATED FOR THEMSELVES

American Psychological Association. "Fat Shaming in the Doctor's Office Can Be Mentally and Physically Harmful: Health Care Providers May Offer Weight Loss Advice in Place of Medical Treatment, Researchers Say." *ScienceDaily*, August 3, 2017. www.sciencedaily.com/releases/2017/08/170803092015.htm.

Bacon, Linda et al. "Size Acceptance and Intuitive Eating Improve Health for Obese, Female Chronic Dieters." *Journal of the American Dietetic Association* 105, no. 6 (2005): 929–36. doi:10.1016/j.jada.2005.03.011.

Carlson, Doug. "Weight Discrimination Linked to Increased Risk of Mortality." *Florida State University News,* October 15, 2015. https://news.fsu.edu/news/health-medicine/2015/10/15/weight-discrimination-linked-to-increased-risk-of-mortality/.

Carter-Kahn, Sophia and April K. Quioh. "Episode 2.5: She's All Fat Goes to the Doctor," March 1, 2018 in *She's All Fat,* produced by Sophie Carter-Khan, podcast, MP3 audio.

Carter-Khan, Sophia. "How to Advocate for Yourself at the Doctor as a Fat Person." *Yahoo! Life,* January 4, 2018, https://www.yahoo.com/lifestyle/advocate-doctor-fat-person-120023980.html.

Mensinger JL, Calogero RM, Stranges S, Tylka TL. "A Weight-Neutral versus Weight-Loss Approach for Health Promotion in Women with High BMI: A Randomized-Controlled Trial." *Appetite.* (2016) 105: no. 364–374. doi:10.1016/j.appet.2016.06.006.

Pidgeon, Elizabeth. "It's 'Lazy Medicine' When Doctors Blame Everything on Your Weight." *The Mighty* (blog), June 18, 2019.

https://themighty.com/2019/06/lazy-medicine-doctors-blaming-health-on-weight-fatphobia/.

CHAPTER 13: WEIGHT MANAGEMENT HAS NO PLACE IN EVIDENCE-BASED CARE

Adams K.M., K.C. Lindell, M. Kohlmeier, S.H. Zeisel. "Status of Nutrition Education in Medical Schools." *Am J Clin Nutr.,* 83, no. 4 (2006): 941S–944S. doi:10.1093/ajcn/83.4.941S.

Harrison, Christy. "Food Psych #207: Doctors Without Diet Culture with Louise Metz," September 30, 2019, in *Food Psych Podcast,* produced by Christy Harrison. Podcast, computer audio, 29:33. https://christyharrison.com/foodpsych/7/doctors-without-diet-culture-with-louise-metz.

Jon Robison. "Health at Every Size: Toward a New Paradigm of Weight and Health." *MedGenMed : Medscape General Medicine,* 7, no. 3, (July 2005): 13, 12.

Made in the USA
Las Vegas, NV
18 January 2021